Inquiries in Bioethics

Inquiries in Bioethics

Stephen G. Post

GEORGETOWN UNIVERSITY PRESS / WASHINGTON, D.C.

Georgetown University Press, Washington, D.C.   20057–1079
© 1993 by Georgetown University Press. All rights reserved.
Printed in the United States of America
10 9 8 7 6 5 4 3 2 1   1993
THIS VOLUME IS PRINTED ON ACID-FREE OFFSET BOOK PAPER.

Library of Congress Cataloging-in-Publication Data

Post, Stephen Garrard, 1951-
    Inquiries in bioethics / Stephen G. Post.
        p.   cm.
    Includes bibliographical references and index.
    1. Medical ethics.   I. Title.
    R724.P665   1993   174'.2--doc   93-17564
    ISBN 0-87840-538-0   ISBN 0-87840-539-9 (pbk.)

Contents

7
Old-Age-Based Rationing, Dementia, and Quality of Life   115

8
The Legacy of Racial Hygiene: Death and Data   141

9
The Emergence of Species Impartiality: A Medical Critique of Biocentrism   161

Index   177

Preface

The field of bioethics is fascinating because it provides an opportunity to encounter great and perennial themes of human moral inquiry, yet with a heightened sense of urgency pressed upon the consciousness of all citizens by the advancing technologies of the life sciences and of health care. New knowledge and technology force us to examine basic questions of human genetic malleability and perfectibility, of moral relations with nonhuman animals and the wider environment, of human reproduction, of the human struggle with mortality and finitude, and of virtually every other significant moral and existential concern that has an impassioned place in the history of the western and non-western mind.

No single book can do more than select themes and topics that are a reflection of the author's interests. Fortunately, the full interdisciplinary scope of the field of bioethics is splendidly presented in the *Encyclopedia of Bioethics,* edited by Warren T. Reich. I have had the opportunity to learn much from Professor Reich in working with him over the past several years, and wish to express my gratitude. Another person who serves as a model of the interdisciplinary approach to bioethics is James M. Gustafson, whose work I have followed since being among his many students a decade ago at the University of Chicago.

The Center for Biomedical Ethics in the School of Medicine at Case Western Reserve University has provided me with sufficient time and stimulation to pursue the thoughts developed in this book. Teaching in a medical school presents the humanities scholar with myriad new problematics. This is always challenging and often fruitful. Much of my interest in bioethics and gerontology results from an invaluable collaboration with Robert H. Binstock, Henry R. Luce, Professor of Aging, Health and Society at Case Western; with Joseph M. Foley, a much admired physician in the field of Alzheimer's disease, and with Peter J. Whitehouse, director of the Alzheimer's Center at University Hospitals of Cleveland.

My wife Mitsuko and my daughter Emma Yoko were very supportive in my work, in understanding the priorities and hopes that engaged me in this endeavor. Thanks to them especially.

STEPHEN G. POST

Acknowledgments

Grateful acknowledgment is made to the editors and publishers for permission to publish those portions of this book that are revisions of previously published articles.

Chapter 1, "Designer Babies, Selective Abortion, and Human Perfection," is a revision of "Selective Abortion and Gene Therapy: Reflections on Human Limits," *Human Gene Therapy* 2, no. 3 (1991): 229–233.

Chapter 2, "The Moral Meaning of Relinquishing an Infant: Reflections on Adoption," is a revision of an article of the same title appearing in *Thought* 67, no. 265 (June 1992): 207–220.

Chapter 3, "Adolescents in Time of AIDS," is a revision of "Adolescents in Time of AIDS: Preventive Education," *America* 167, no. 11 (October 1992): 278–282.

Chapter 4, "Psychiatry and the Challenge of Religious Toleration," is a revision of "Psychiatry, Religious Conversion and Bioethics," *Kennedy Institute of Ethics Journal* 1, no. 3 (March 1991): 207–223.

Chapter 5, "American Culture and Good Death," is a revision of "American Culture and Euthanasia," *Health Progress* 72, no. 10 (December 1991): 32–39. The article was awarded second place by the Catholic Press Association of the United States and Canada for "best article originating with a professional journal" in 1991.

Chapter 6, "The Covenant of Basic Caring," is previously unpublished, but some of its ideas are taken from "Family Caretaking: Stewardship and Commitment," *Second Opinion: Health, Faith, and Ethics* 8 (July 1988): 114–127.

Chapter 8, "The Legacy of Racial Hygiene: Death and Data," is a revision of "The Legacy of Racial Hygiene: Hearing the Voice of Victims," *Soundings: An Interdisciplinary Journal* 74 nos. 3 and 4 (Fall/Winter 1991): 541–558.

Chapter 9, "The Emergence of Species Impartiality: A Medical Critique of Biocentrism," is a revision of an article of the same title previously published in *Perspectives in Biology and Medicine* 36, no. 2 (1993): 289–300.

Introduction

Bioethics is an interdisciplinary field concerned with issues in the life sciences, health, and health care. In this book I explore nine representative bioethical issues loosely organized in a sequence from birth and youth to aging and death. I have drawn on the insights of religious studies, history, philosophy, and health care in order to develop broad perspectives for an interdisciplinary readership. My method is shaped by no overarching foundational moral theory, although general principles such as "do no harm" (nonmaleficence) are presumed. I attempt to present perspectives in the tradition of the public intellectual concerned that too much work in bioethics is overly theory-driven and intended for specialized peer groups. My attention to a spectrum of broad, perennial, humanistic themes such as human perfectibility, trust, care, and the contingency of human experience will, I hope, prove engaging and possibly refreshing. Throughout the book I place emphasis on the cultural changes that underlie and shape our presuppositions about the right and the good. In the end, the reader will rightfully detect that I am not a consistent defender of modernity.

The biological revolution that is currently taking place, with its attendant technological powers to alter nature and human nature, requires of all thoughtful people a fundamental and cautionary reflection on questions of the highest ethical importance. In the first chapter, "Designer Babies, Selective Abortion, and Human Perfection," I raise serious questions about the advent of new magnitudes of genetic knowledge that can narrow parental images of human normalcy in a culture prone to forget that what human perfection is available to us is, as Aristotle understood, largely a matter of good character forged in response to the lessons of experience. Our eyes wrongly turn toward the appearance of the human vessel rather than to the virtues of the person. That almighty data replace the mystery of the womb is a mixed blessing and, increasingly, a cultural mandate.

My defense, in chapter 2, of relinquishing an infant for the benefit of childless couples who wish to experience parenthood will disturb some critics who exaggerate the harms this practice inflicts on the child. In response to anticipated criticism, I consider these alleged harms in a balanced manner in the first section of the chapter. I propose greater moral emphasis on the value of relinquishing a child for adoption as an idealistic alternative to abortion. Such idealism, however, neither can nor should be required. The relinquishing of a child by the biological mother has in our current culture been denigrated, in distinct contrast to earlier historical periods in which it was understood more positively. We have something to learn from this history.

Chapter 3, "Adolescents in Time of AIDS," is a shift from birth ethics to a tragic epidemic that threatens the young, and about which all parents are concerned as they see their children growing up. The Committee on Adolescence of the American Academy of Pediatrics issued a report entitled "Contraception and Adolescents" in 1990. The report deserves more attention than it has received. It is noteworthy first for its opening directive that pediatricians should be "active participants in the effort to reduce the negative consequences of adolescent sexual activity." The second sentence is this: "Preventive measures include counseling teenagers and their families on responsible sexual decisionmaking, including abstinence, and providing contraceptive services for sexually active patients, when requested." Throughout the report, a special concern is with the transmission of the human immunodeficiency virus (HIV), in response to which pediatricians are to encourage patients to "postpone first intercourse until they are physiologically and psychologically mature."[1] Throughout, the pediatrician is to remain nonjudgmental and nonthreatening. This support for prevention is grounded in the experiences of pediatricians who have witnessed the huge impact of infectious diseases from *Chlamydia trachomatis* and *Treponema pallidum* to herpes simplex virus and HIV. Pediatricians seem able to transcend our various "culture wars" regarding sexual morality in order to focus on the one value that every citizen shares, especially with regard to young lives, the avoidance of disease and death. Because this issue is increasingly significant for parents and children, it is a fit area for serious ethical discussion.

Some theories of moral development suggest that adolescents and young adults often go through a phase in which they quest for an absolute and all-encompassing worldview. Sociologists, among them Peter Berger, emphasize the psychic burden of growing up in a modern culture with many competing worldviews that relativize all assertions about ultimate reality. Uprooted and traditionless, the "homeless mind" struggles to find meaning in modernity, often migrating from worldview to worldview in a search for the one and only truth. It is remarkable how many of my peers in the 1970s and 1980s joined rigorous and in some cases relatively authoritarian political, social, or religious movements only to pass through the revolving door of utopianism back into the world, generally a bit wiser for the experience. Migrations into the more radical religious movements stirred particular controversy among their parents and attracted wide attention from psychiatrists. In chapter 4, "Psychiatry and the Challenge of Religious Toleration," I discuss ethics, psychiatry, and parental response to socially unaccepted ideological movements. I deal with the so-called "deprogramming" controversy, as parents attempt to rescue their young adult children from intense organizations, sometimes with assistance from psychiatrists and often unaware of the extraordinarily high attrition rates that naturally occur in these organizations as naïveté gives rise to suspicion. I review literature from the American Psychiatric Association in the light of a wider discussion of modernity, family interests, and anomie. This chapter is dedicated to my old friend Jake, whom I met while a college student. Jake migrated through no less than three intense religious movements between 1970 and 1974 before settling into a tree house in the forests of Oregon to find his own truth. He is now an insightful anti-utopian and a Catholic.

The end of youth might be defined as the dawning of our sense of finitude and our desire to leave behind something meaningful in the time allotted to us. A central bioethical concern is the human response to the temporal limits imposed by our biological embeddedness. One of the perennial questions in all cultures is how to respond morally to inevitable bodily and very often mental decline. In the last analysis, a divide separates those who would strike out against this decline by preemptive suicide or voluntary mercy killing and those who prefer to leave the hour of their deaths in the hands of nature or of nature's God. I discuss these issues in chapter 5, "American Culture and Good Death." Of course, those who wish no preemptive suicide may require considerable care and attention from loved ones or other care givers. Thus, the issues considered in the sixth chapter, "The Covenant of Basic Caring," are linked with those in chapter 5.

In these two chapters, I avoid the words "active euthanasia" and "passive euthanasia" because they suggest two instances of what is more or less the same action. It is better to speak of killing and allowing to die, emphasizing a moral difference between aiming to end a life and removing treatments in the knowledge that if the patient continues to live he or she will be cared for steadfastly. In the second instance, if the patient dies, the result is the same as killing, but what the physician *does* and *becomes* as an intentional moral agent is very different.

In chapter 6 I provide an alternative to suicide and killing. A hospice physician, David Cundiff, notes that requests for mercy killing are uncommon according to polls of cancer specialists. What requests are made stem from poor pain control and/or inadequate psychosocial support. Those who make requests "almost always change their minds once their physical symptoms are controlled and they are placed in a caring, supportive, hospice environment." Cundiff's thesis is that "vastly improved hospice training for health care professionals, along with better quality and greater availability of hospice services can render the issues of euthanasia and assisted suicide essentially moot."[2] There is much to be said for the hospice viewpoint, or so I will argue.

In chapter 7, "Old-Age-Based Rationing, Dementia, and Quality of Life," I discuss preemptive suicide in cases of irreversible dementias in addition to providing criticism of the rationing of health care based on age. Alzheimer's disease is on the cutting edge of the national and international debate about physician-assisted suicide. While it is true that requests for suicide from the terminally ill are often shaped by untreated pain and inadequate psychosocial conditions, what of requests by people with diagnoses of progressive dementia that will ultimately lead to the loss of memory and hence of self-identity, and a decline over as many as fifteen years? Such cases are beyond the beneficent hand of hospice care. Reports consistently indicate that in the Netherlands, where assisted suicide and mercy killing are de facto accepted, about 10 percent of requests come from patients with chronic degenerative neurological disorders.[3] Margaret P. Battin writes of progressive dementia: "This is the condition the Dutch call *entluistering*, the 'effacement' or complete eclipse of human personality, and for the Dutch, *entluistering* rather than pain is a primary reason for choices of [active] euthanasia."[4] Battin defends assisted suicide or mercy killing in cases of progressive dementia if requested by a living will or by personal directive. I make no such defense but instead offer a compromise.

The eighth chapter, "The Legacy of Racial Hygiene: Death and Data," is about a time when medicine became murderous. The art of medicine slipped deeply into the habit of killing, and no discussion of the ethics of death is complete without recollecting this. I have in mind the incredible human destruction at the hands of the Nazi doctors. Whether the Nazi period has much analogical significance for the current discussion over assisted suicide and medical killing is unclear and a matter of continuing debate. Still, it is important to remind ourselves of this history.

Finally, in the last chapter, entitled "The Emergence of Species Impartiality: A Medical Critique of Biocentrism," I raise an underlying moral question: is a human life more important than any nonhuman animal's, even when that animal is relatively highly evolved? In a well-publicized case in 1992, Dr. Thomas E. Starzl transplanted a baboon liver into a thirty-five-year-old man who died seventy-one days later after a stroke. The case presents an opportunity for debate between those who would save a human life at the sacrifice of a baboon, and those who find such salvation morally disgraceful. Because human cruelty toward members of nonhuman species has occurred throughout history, it may be good that interspecies egalitarianism has emerged. Yet does interspecies egalitarianism leave us with a deeply distorted model of our proper rights and obligations? Many observers may question the particular choice of patient or other clinical-ethical aspects of Starzl's liver transplants. But Starzl has acted on the moral assumption that the human good remains appropriately the highest good, despite the cultural inroads of anthropomorphism.

NOTES

1. Committee on Adolescence, American Academy of Pediatrics, "Contraception and Adolescents," *Pediatrics* 86, no. 1 (July 1990): 134.

2. See David Cundiff, *Euthanasia Is Not the Answer: A Hospice Physician's View* (Totowa, New Jersey: Humana Press, 1992), p. 16.

3. Maurice A. M. de Wachter, "Euthanasia in the Netherlands," *Hastings Center Report* 22, no. 2 (March–April 1992): 23–30.

4. Margaret P. Battin, "Euthanasia in Alzheimer's Disease?" in Robert H. Binstock, Stephen G. Post, and Peter J. Whitehouse, eds., *Dementia and Aging: Ethics, Values and Policy Choices* (Baltimore: Johns Hopkins University Press, 1992), p. 123.

1

Designer Babies, Selective Abortion, and Human Perfection

The project to map and sequence the human genome is under way. The number of gene abnormalities that can be tested for will dramatically increase from several hundred to many more within the decade and perhaps to thousands.[1] Prenatal, neonatal, carrier, and presymptomatic testing will reach new orders of magnitude.[2] Such testing will remain a matter of personal choice in our highly individualistic culture, unless restricted by health care rationing or some other aspect of social and distributive justice. Nevertheless, even if the individual has a legal right to any and all testing he or she can afford, there is room for moral discussion of the broad humanistic foundations of the choices that individuals will be making about selective abortion on the basis of genetic defects.

Lest this essay be misinterpreted, I must state immediately that those opposed to abortion should not, for that reason, frown on the human genome project to map chromosomally, or locate, all human genes. The emerging technology of somatic cell gene therapy will possibly provide an alternative for parents who might otherwise resort to selective abortion. Eve K. Nichols suggests a scenario in which prenatal diagnosis detects severe combined immune deficiency. Knowing of the disease in advance, physicians could prepare a germ-free "bubble" environment for the baby. Then, the adenosine deaminase gene could be inserted into the baby's bone marrow cells. This autologous transplant would result in normal lymphocytes, and in a healthy child.[3] While we must not exaggerate the possibilities for human gene therapy, which is still largely speculative, possible future scenarios such as Nichols's indicate that the genome project should not be captured by the politics of antiabortion. Many severe and early-onset diseases for which selective abortion would now be morally justified may be treatable through gene transfer in future decades.

SEVERITY, PROBABILITY, AND AGE AT ONSET OF DISEASE

Although selective abortion is an old topic, the genome project raises it in a newly important way. Most Americans accept prenatal diagnosis and subsequent abortion for grave or relatively serious genetic defects that would manifest early in the sufferer's life. They are critical, however, of termination of pregnancy for trivial or moderately serious genetic defects and for defects that would appear only later in life.[4] Given the legal right to elective abortion, of which the right to selective abortion is a subset, it is wise to consider the moral underpinnings of the choices that women and couples are free to make.

I am concerned here with selective abortions for less severe diseases and for those which appear in mid-life or later. Although such abortions are largely a *potential* problem at present, an old Jewish aphorism, "Start worrying, letter to follow!" seems applicable. For now, such prenatal testing for late-onset diseases is not readily available except for a few cases, including Huntington's chorea, and it is not clear that large numbers of people would want to have such tests.

The problem is *largely* potential but not entirely so. Barbara Katz Rothman provides a number of case studies in which abortion was chosen as an alternative to mild diseases and to impairments that were less than disabling. She suggests a future in which we will see emerging from new technologies "a rise in the standards of production for children." She asks if we will "establish a set of norms of acceptability, and then narrow, and narrow, and narrow yet again those norms?"[5]

In response to this potential problem, Dorothy C. Wetz and John C. Fletcher, supporters of the genome project, argue that the medical profession should abandon a position of ethical neutrality with regard to prenatal sex selection, partly because it sets precedents for selection unrelated to disease or disability, for example, for eye and hair color, thinness, skin color, straight teeth, and other "cosmetic" considerations. Within a decade or two, they continue, these "exotic" choices will be technically possible, especially those relating to body size and height.[6]

Prenatal testing will eventually be capable of detecting hundreds or thousands of single gene defects, many more polygenic and multifactorial defects, and numerous superficial characteristics of aesthetic concern. Experts believe that pregnant women, at about eight to ten weeks gestation, may soon be able to have a blood test indicating the DNA profile of the fetus based on fetal cells in the maternal circulation. This extensive new level of knowledge leads to tremendously complex personal choices about what lives are worth living, qualitatively considered.[7]

That women have the unlimited legal right to choose abortion is a fact of American culture, but here is where the discussion begins in regard to personal moral conscience. In the absence of an obviously grave and immediately threatening defect, vexing decisions will be made based on severity, probability, and age at onset of disease or disability. Turner's syndrome, for instance, affects girls, resulting in shortness, infertility, and often odd appearance (for example, a web neck). Still, life expectancy is normal, and with in vitro fertilization it has become possible for some of those suffering from Turner's syndrome to have babies. Probability of occurrence is clear, as is age at onset, but the severity of the syndrome might not be considered great. The difficulty, ethically, comes with parental decisions about the acceptability of the child's quality of life. Another example would be polycystic kidney disease, which may or may not occur and which results in progressive renal failure during the adult years. It is, of course, treatable by dialysis or transplant. In this example, moderate severity combines with uncertainty of manifestation and late onset. Huntington's chorea can be distinguished from polycystic kidney disease because it is much more severe and untreatable. Would an abortion be morally justifiable for a fetus if the future child had a 20 percent probability of bipolar affective disorder? What about cystic fibrosis, Duchenne type muscular dystrophy, blindness, or familial Alzheimer's disease? What shall we do with the freedom to decide, especially when genetic conditions have variable expression from mild to serious, have variable likelihood of manifestation, are variable as to age at onset, and may be treatable?

At a minimum, we can distinguish moral from aesthetic values and give priority to the former. Is a disease such as Huntington's chorea insufficient grounds for selective abortion because, even though it is clearly very severe, the eventual sufferer nevertheless will have many decades of good and unimpaired living? Moreover, the parents of the child are not immediately or necessarily directly affected in the way they would be were the disease of early onset.

I do not want to go very far in resolving the balance between severity, probability, and age at onset that might for many justify selective abortion. Rather, I offer several humanistic reflections to provide a general background for such decisions; together they justify reservations at least about abortions for diseases that appear later in life or are of lesser severity. My limited intention is to comment on American culture, focusing on three themes: the parental desire to avoid bringing suffering into the world; the contingencies of the human condition; and the deep moral ambiguity of the quest for "perfect" babies. These themes will be linked both to selective abortion and, more briefly, to gene therapy.

THE SUFFERING OF OFFSPRING

Parents rightfully prefer not to bring lives filled with suffering into the world. Few, if any, would quarrel with the assumption that it is preferable to have healthy children who are not born into physical pain. When pre-natal diagnosis reveals a grave defect that makes life an onerous burden of suffering, the principle "do no harm" may for many but certainly not all parents morally justify abortion. But it is wrong to assume that suffering is the necessary result of every genetic defect, or that lives with degrees of physical suffering cannot be creative and meaningful. Moreover, human beings are finite creatures thrown into suffering, from which there is no ultimate escape. We confront our frailties sooner or later, and much of human enlightenment is to know that even in brokenness there is hope. That suffering and the necessity of meeting its challenge creatively is a universal existential predicament seems perfectly obvious. In this sense, placing all hope in a genetic response to suffering is, finally, misplaced. Still, suffering can and should be mitigated when possible, rather than be viewed positively.

Certainly some individuals compensate for "imperfections" through living exceptionally creative and highly productive lives. They can tolerate their challenges rather well. Fyodor Dostoyevsky, for instance, suffered from seizure disorder. In a letter to the famous critic Nikolai Strakhov, he wrote these remarkable words: "For a few moments before the fit, I experience a feeling of happiness such as it is quite impossible to imagine in a normal state and which other people have no idea of. I feel entirely in harmony with myself and the whole world, and this feeling is so strong and so delightful that for a few seconds of such bliss one would gladly give up ten years of one's life, if not one's whole life."[8] This passage is a powerful indication that there can be less suffering present in the experience of an illness than might be supposed. Quality of life is never a matter for purely objective measurement; it always contains some subjective element, except in the most severe circumstances of neurological impairment. Quality of life is in part a self-fulfilling prophecy; that is, we create an environment that precludes quality of life for the person with a disability because we do not believe that quality is possible, although it is.

Adrienne Asch, an advocate of rights for disabled persons, herself blind and a professor at a major university, points out that as prenatal diagnosis results in vast new genetic knowledge, women need "to obtain far more and very different information than they very commonly get about people with disabilities."[9] The notion that all disabilities cause suffering is conceptually flawed. In many cases, negative stereotypes obscure the creative ways in which people with disabilities can live their lives.

The genome project calls for scrutiny of the assumption that those who are different from what society considers normal necessarily suffer. Our societal inclination to rather narrow standards of beauty, physical prowess, and self-reliance prompt us too easily to assume that those who fall short of these standards therefore suffer and even deserve our compassion.

With respect to human gene therapy, the principle of beneficence provides sufficient moral justification "to use somatic cell gene therapy for treatment of serious disease."[10] As long as gene therapy is limited to inherited disorders that result from the absence of gene products, no one would reasonably object to it. The analogy is to organ transplantation, but on the cellular level. It is possible that our cultural definitions of normalcy might shift so that genetic engineering with the goal of enhancement of the human being becomes increasingly attractive. The therapeutic repair of human beings is noble, but efforts to enhance the already healthy are inherently problematic. What defines enhancement? Are taller and more slender people better? And where would the endless so-called enhancement end? When everyone is an inch taller, then what? Serious and objective medical need, rather than the vicissitudes of enhancement, is the proper basis for genetic interventions. Regrettably, the line between therapy and enhancement is not always clear. The possibility for confusion between human wants and genuine human needs is real. A parent may want a "designer" child via gene enhancement, but this is not something that parent or child needs.

The desire to eliminate disease and the sufferings that may be associated with illness is morally valid. The definition of suffering, however, is wrongly expanded to include the ways in which an individual is different from others. Suffering becomes a social construct imposed on us, so that parents will petition the physician to "enhance" a child regardless of the folly of the request. It is incumbent on physicians to hold firmly against the quest for enhancement, in part by maintaining a disease-based definition of the human suffering for which medical therapy is responsible for alleviating. To widen the definition of suffering so as to provide enhancement interventions is precisely the wrong response to the human condition. Moreover, such interventions violate the purpose of the healing art, which is the restoration of physical and mental function when possible, or else comfort care and the control of pain.[11]

CONTINGENCY AND CONTROL

Throughout human history every mother and father has lived with the mystery of the womb. Many prayed to God or the gods and goddesses that the fruits of the womb might be whole and unimperiled. The word "contingency" refers to a chance event beyond control, and this all births were. Our desire not to bring imperfection into the world must be tempered by a recognition that suffering brought about by events we can never control is an ineradicable part of life. Those who are genotypically and phenotypically more "perfect" than others can lead tragic lives, brought about by unforeseen circumstances. Take the case of the great French artist Henri de Toulouse-Lautrec. A descendent of aristocrats, he was the victim of two accidents that broke his legs and left him incurably disabled. His torso developed but not his legs, and he became deformed, unable to walk without a cane. He derived some consolation from painting, until dipsomania led to the asylum.

His was an irregular life, one of immense suffering; it was also one of creative compensation and the development of the artistic poster as we know it today. Lautrec was born a normal infant, for all intents and purposes a perfect baby. But the contingencies of human experience that range from accident to bad luck left him disabled anyway. His diminutive stature both caused him suffering and simultaneously may have elevated him artistically, although it is erroneous to suggest that disabilities necessarily give rise to unusual forms of creativity as a compensatory response.[12]

As for the effort to remove contingency from human experience, technological culture encourages ever greater control over what was once left to chance or mystery. Yet chance is at the very heart of human experience. An ancient Taoist text, about the old man and the horse, is instructive. There was an old man who had a horse, the story goes. One day the horse ran away. The neighbors came and said "Old man, old man, how unfortunate." He responded, "How do you know?" The next day, the horse returned with two other wild horses beside it. The neighbors said, "Old man, old man, how fortunate." "How do you know?" he answered. His beloved son went riding on one of the new stallions, which threw him, breaking his leg. The neighbors said, "Old man, old man, how unfortunate." He responded, "How do you know?" At that time, as it turned out, many young men were being drafted into a work force to build the great wall of China. Most of them died. The old man's son was too crippled to go. The neighbors said, "Old man, old man, how fortunate." His only answer was, "How do you know?"

This story expresses the extent to which we cannot control events nor easily predict what joys or sufferings will flow from them. The classical prescientific Western culture left events largely in the hands of a mysterious deity whose ultimate purposes were presumed to be loving. Does technology foster a rage to control and thus prevent our coming to grips with the basic reality of contingency from which we never escape?

No matter how much we attempt control, suffering is a part of all human lives, to greater or lesser degrees.[13] The Tantric Buddhist will state that if you are born, you will suffer; life is understood as suffering unto growth, until the wheel of rebirth is finally escaped. Indeed, transformative suffering is viewed as the only point of human bodily existence.

Contingency, lack of control, is the chief source of what existentialist philosophers and theologians have dubbed anxiety, following Kierkegaard. To be out of control is discomforting, and from it emerges the desire to dominate both nature and human nature. But, of course, human finitude has the last word: we are finally under the essential control of the nature that is destiny, complete with massive epidemics. We must come to grips with the human predicament; we need worldviews that firmly capture the fact of contingency. Human beings are finite, bounded creatures subject to countless contingencies, and with very little final control.

PERFECTION

The right of only so-called perfect babies to exist is not a matter of public policy, but each time a selective abortion for a moderate or trivial imperfection occurs, we are in effect accepting this principle. Gradually, society moves perilously closer to Nietzsche's norm: "The weak and ill-constituted shall perish: first principle of *our* philanthropy. And one shall help them to do so."[14]

All perfectionism must be tempered by an awareness of what Leslie A. Fiedler calls "the tyranny of the normal."[15] Fiedler notes a "deep ambivalence toward fellow creatures who are perceived at any given moment as disturbingly deviant, outside currently acceptable physiological norms."[16] He refers to "a vestigial primitive fear of the abnormal, exacerbated by guilt." Fiedler fears the "enforced physiological normalcy" that sent dwarfs to extermination camps in Hitler's Germany. "Perhaps it is especially important for us to realize that finally there are no normals, at a moment when we are striving desperately to eliminate freaks, to normalize the world."[17]

One of the ways in which persons who depart from "normals" contribute to the community is by challenging us to overcome social stigmas and to accept difference in our midst. Views of physiological human perfection are inevitably intertwined with stigmas, one form of which is "abominations" of the body.[18] Those whose bodies depart negatively from the "normals" are the victims of a socially shaped tendency to revulsion. Stigmas specific to the body are as morally problematic as those related to religion, race, and nationality and often cause great suffering to disabled people. People who are different and "imperfect" teach us about the meaning of equality and commitment. But we are beings who fear difference, so diversity is hard to sustain.

The very nature of human perfection has, of course, been the subject of acrimonious debate over the centuries. In the medieval period, there was a profound sense that perfection is chiefly a matter of character and virtue and that bodily imperfections provide opportunities for concentration on the internal moral and spiritual values. Indeed, the weight of religious symbolism, from the clubfooted Christ figure of the Eastern Orthodox icons to Dostoyevsky's epileptic savior, underscores the inward perfection made possible by external limitations. What human perfection can be approximated is finally characterological.

There is treasure in earthen vessels, and earthen vessels we humans are, subject to countless infections, accidents, chronic ailments, and finally to the decline of old age and death that we in this culture try so hard to deny, as though senility were mere myth. Arguably, our culture focuses perfection on the vessel rather than on the person within it, however dualistic this may sound. Of course it is reasonable to avoid bringing grave human imperfection into the world, especially when an infant will have no potential to relate to other human beings. But we must be highly circumspect about declaring too imperfect those who must endure early in life the very sorts of frailties that eventually assault each one of us.

It is especially ill conceived when a society so overvalues beauty and physical prowess that ugliness and bodily weakness are aborted out of existence. Aesthetic vicissitudes might increasingly determine who should, and who should not, inhabit the world.[19] But this determination is fundamentally flawed (the Buddha would laugh). It is rooted in mistaken attachments to the bodily vessel of the human self, and not to the self in its essence. Arguably, our culture is pitifully narrow in the externality of its perfectionism.

Our medical system, with its relentless drive to fix and rescue, reinforces the ideal and possibility of human perfection, but perfection is a highly elusive notion that allows for no simple definitions. The very ability to reach into the human genome creates by anticipation some vague image of perfection constitutive of progress. But we must be wary of images and enthusiasms that are poorly considered. In particular, enhancement and eugenic genetic engineering are problematic because they tend to further externalize our images of human perfection and do not result in any clear moral good. By externalized perfection I mean definitions of the human good that are centered on the shape of the body, or on some particular capacity for music, visual arts, and so forth. All the major cultures of the world, with the help of religious worldviews, have defined human perfection internally, that is, with emphasis on character and virtue. From Aristotle to Thomas Aquinas, perfection meant wisdom rooted in experience and in the relationships by which the moral life is learned through example.

CULTURAL CHANGE

It might seem farfetched that selective abortion would be chosen based on susceptibility to disease in the distant future, or on a "cosmetic" basis, "but social mores change rapidly in the face of new technology."[20] Prenatal testing may encompass everything from eventual susceptibility to colon cancer, to musicianship or height. As it has been put, "Our increasing ability to control our reproduction and to determine prenatally the genetic endowment of our children changes both the practice of medicine and the concept of humanness."[21] Whether, with vast new genetic knowledge, our reproductive lives, our tolerance of difference, and our communities will be better off still remains to be seen.

There is no reason for undue pessimism. The broad cultural questions raised by prenatal testing and selective abortion are obviously relevant to gene therapy itself. As William F. Anderson writes, "At the core of society's concern about beginning the human application of genetic engineering may be our sense that we are developing a capability to *change* who and what we are."[22] Human beings, particularly in a secular and technological age, have need for what I will call *object consciousness,* that is, the sense that they are formed and situated under the guise of a subject with wisdom greater than their own. When, in endless individualism, they seek to climb the mast that they might recreate themselves or their children beyond therapeutic boundaries, the ship leans one way and then the other to the point of finally capsizing.

All of this said, I see moral value in the genome project. Tests for a high predisposition for colorectal cancer years before the disease strikes would allow predisposed people to modify their lifestyle in a healthful and preventive manner. Potential cures through somatic cell gene therapy may emerge for diseases of genetic etiology. Selective abortions, which are not desired in the same way that elective abortions are, might be avoided through gene therapy. Most of all, the genome project challenges society to reflect deeply on what makes a life worth bringing into the world, and what sorts of uses of medical interventions, consistent with the limits of the human condition, are justified.

Women have the legal right to choose abortion, whatever one might think about it. Room is still left, however, for discussion of the moral considerations that might inform individual conscience as this right is exercised. I also have no interest in questioning selective abortion for grave genetic defects that will manifest immediately or early in life. Selective abortion for trivial or moderately serious genetic defects, and for diseases that will manifest later in life, however, raises serious moral concern.

Conditions that appear in adulthood, such as Huntington's chorea, raise perplexing questions. Huntington's usually manifests between the ages of thirty and fifty. It is clearly a severe disease, even insidious. Personality changes, choreic movements, paranoid reactions, cognitive impairment, and dementia are just some of the phenomena that occur. The illness can last for a decade or slightly more, resulting eventually in death. L. M. Purdy writes thus: "For devastating diseases like Huntington's chorea, this part of the judgment should be unproblematic: no one would want a loved one to suffer so."[23] Certainly not. Still, I dispute Purdy's argument that, from the potential child's point of view, it is unethical not to abort. The child, he claims, deserves an "opportunity for a good life."

Contra Purdy, I assert that a life of thirty to fifty years duration is potentially a fully good one. The meanings and experiences that so many years afford could easily surpass those who live to old age but lived purposelessly. The suffering brought on by Huntington's chorea as symptoms manifest is severe but not categorically more so than is the case with the dementias that afflict many elderly people. Preemptive suicide, while not something I would defend, may yet become an option (see chapter 7).[24]

It is morally presumptuous to argue that from the child's perspective, life with Huntington's chorea is wrongful. Of course parents have a legal right to abort in the case of prenatal genetic detection of Huntington's chorea. I only contend that, ethically, the grounds for such abortions are at least questionable. Parents want to avoid bringing suffering into the world, but they can never fully accomplish this to begin with, as I have argued previously. Parents want "perfect babies," but how does one measure perfection, and what levels of fulfillment are open to those who may be eventual victims of diseases that appear in mid-life or later?

My intent has been to raise questions about selective abortion for even severe late-onset diseases. There is, of course, room for conscientious disagreement in most ethical debates. Abortion for Huntington's chorea, however, is not easily justified.

The same can be said with regard to Alzheimer's disease, the most common cause of dementia. Unlike Huntington's chorea, the genetics of Alzheimer's disease are still being researched. Yet, "because of growing evidence for genetic causes of Alzheimer's disease, clinicians are often asked about risks for this disorder among relatives of patients."[25]

The aspect of Alzheimer's disease that makes it problematic with respect to selective abortion is its late onset. Certainly if the onset were very early in life, familial Alzheimer's disease might be analogous to Tay-Sachs disease, with the progressive neurologic decline of a child being a major burden to parents. But the decades of unaffected life in Alzheimer's disease force us to carefully assess the burden of the disease on both the person and his or her parents.

Pregnancy termination for Alzheimer's disease cannot be clearly construed as beneficial to the fetus. The effect on the quality of life of the individual is variable and he or she has the prospects of as many as five decades of unimpaired life. In addition, it is critical to recognize that the elucidation of the genetic basis for the disease that permits prenatal testing may also permit an intervention—amelioration, if not a cure—within the decades prior to disease onset. Thus, it is difficult to mount a convincing argument that the fetus would choose termination given his or her risk of future Alzheimer's disease.

The perspective of the parents may be different from that envisioned for the fetus. Does the burden of bearing a child destined to have Alzheimer's disease justify selective abortion? It has been argued that "the judgment of poor quality of life may be made by the one who lives the life or by an observer. It often happens that lives which observers consider of poor quality are lived quite satisfactorily by the one living that life."[26]

The key question is, Is it morally acceptable to terminate a pregnancy because of the risk of Alzheimer's disease, Huntington's chorea, or other diseases that appear in adulthood? Abortion does not seem to promote the welfare of the child in any obvious sense. Further, it does not obviously promote the interests of the parents, given the contingency of the human condition generally. The future disease of the child will not necessarily place tangible burdens on them. If dementia strikes the individual as an adult, then the burdens of care can be shared by spouses, friends, and society more broadly. I do not intend to diminish the suffering that parents may feel in the illness and decline of an adult child, but I question whether by itself the speculative anticipation of distant future suffering justifies the termination of a fetus.

Finally, every woman or couple decide for themselves how much fine-tuning of the lives and life spans of their children is justifiable. Alzheimer's disease seems to me to exemplify the moral limits of fine-tuning. Another valid concern is that selective abortion for Alzheimer's disease would establish an excessive standard of control over the genetic nature of the fetus.

In the area of genetic testing for purposes of possible selective abortion, the debate two decades old began over severe and immediate onset conditions such as Down's syndrome. Some critics argued that once selective abortion was in place for immediate and early-onset diseases, the practice would expand to include trivial abnormalities and diseases of later onset. In the event that selective abortions for late-onset diseases become widespread, the critics will have been right; the "slippery slope" will in this instance have been real. The argument that once prenatal genetic testing and selective abortion get a foot in the culture's door they can only proceed to their full extreme may yet be verified. This is reason for pause. How much selective abortion is enough?

NOTES

1. National Research Council Committee on Mapping and Sequencing the Human Genome, *Mapping and Sequencing the Human Genome* (Washington, D.C.: National Academy Press, 1988).

2. Jeffrey R. Botkin, "Ethical Issues in Human Genetic Technology," *Pediatrician* 17 (1990): 100–117.

3. Eve K. Nichols, *Human Gene Therapy: Institute of Medicine/National Academy of Sciences* (Cambridge: Harvard University Press, 1988), p. 2.

4. John A. Robertson, "Procreative Liberty and Human Genetics," *Emory Law Journal* 39 (1990): 697–719.

5. Barbara Katz Rothman, *The Tentative Pregnancy: Prenatal Diagnosis and the Future of Motherhood* (New York: Penguin Books, 1986), p. 227.

6. Dorothy C. Wetz and John C. Fletcher, "Fatal Knowledge? Prenatal Diagnosis and Sex Selection," *Hastings Center Report* 19, no. 3 (1989): 21–27.

7. Diana Frank and Marta Vogel, *The Baby Makers* (New York: Carroll and Graf, 1988).

8. Fyodor Dostoyevsky, *The Idiot*, trans. and with an introduction by David G. Magarshack (New York: Penguin, 1955 [original 1870]), p. 8.

9. Adrienne Asch, "Can Aborting 'Imperfect' Children Be Immoral?" in John Arras and Nancy Rhoden, eds., *Ethical Issues in Modern Medicine* (Mountain View, Calif.: Mayfield Publishing, 1989), p. 320.

10. William F. Anderson, "Genetics and Human Malleability," *Hastings Center Report* 20, no. 1 (1990): 21–24.

11. Leon R. Kass, *Toward a More Natural Science: Biology and Human Affairs* (New York: Free Press, 1985).

12. Thomas Craven, *A Treasury of Art Masterpieces* (New York: Simon and Schuster, 1939), p. 518.

13. Stanley Hauerwas, *Suffering Presence* (Notre Dame, Ind.: University of Notre Dame Press, 1986).

14. Friedrich Nietzsche, *Twilight of the Idols / The Anti-Christ*, trans. R. L. Hollingdale (New York: Penguin, 1978 [original 1895]), p. 116.

15. Leslie A. Fiedler, "The Tyranny of the Normal," in T. H. Murray and A. L. Caplan, eds., *Which Babies Shall Live? Humanistic Dimensions of the Care of Imperiled Newborns* (Clifton, N.J.: Humana Press, 1985), p. 151.

16. Ibid., p. 152.

17. Ibid., p. 157.

18. Erving Goffman, *Stigma: Notes on the Management of Spoiled Identity* (New York: Simon and Schuster, 1986).

19. H. P. Holmes, B. B. Hoskins, and M. Gross, eds., *The Custom-Made Child: Women-Centered Perspectives* (Clifton, N.J.: Humana Press, 1981).

20. J. E. Bishop and M. Waldholz, *Genome* (New York: Simon and Schuster, 1990), p. 20.

21. S. Elias and G. J. Annas, *Reproductive Genetics and the Law* (Chicago: Year Book Medical Publishers, 1987), p. xi.

22. William F. Anderson, "Human Gene Therapy: Why Draw a Line?" *Journal of Medicine and Philosophy* 14 (1989): 682.

23. L. M. Purdy, "Genetic Diseases: Can Having Children Be Immoral?" in R. Munson, ed., *Intervention and Reflection: Basic Issues in Medical Ethics* (Belmont, Calif.: Wadsworth Press, 1992), p. 430.

24. C. G. Prado, *The Last Choice: Preemptive Suicide in Advanced Age* (Westport, Conn.: Greenwood Press, 1990).

25. J. C. S. Brelmer, "Clinical Genetics and Genetic Counseling in Alzheimer Disease," *Annals of Internal Medicine* 115 (1991): 601.

26. A. R. Jonsen, M. Siegler, and W. J. Winslade, *Clinical Ethics* (New York: Macmillan, 1982), p. 111.

2

The Moral Meaning of Relinquishing an Infant: Reflections on Adoption

The focus of this chapter is on adoption viewed from the perspective of the birth mother who relinquishes her infant. Questions about the high cost of adoption and the criteria for adoptive parents are among many not addressed here. Inquiry is limited to the moral considerations that might encourage a birth mother to relinquish her infant, presuming that adoptive parents are caring and committed to their adopted children. To my knowledge, this line of inquiry has been omitted from the current ethics literature.

I am aware of the psychological literature indicating that some adopted children are more vulnerable to certain psychological and school-related problems. Children must cope with the fact that their birth mother relinquished them and that this distinguishes them from their nonadopted counterparts. Yet as one leading expert emphasizes, "it is clear that adopted children display a wide range of adjustment patterns, with only a minority presenting evidence of clinically significant symptomatology. Indeed, most adopted children appear to cope well with the challenges, conflicts, and demands of adoptive family life."[1] Moreover, a systematic empirical study of long-term maladjustment indicates that adoptees are no different from nonadoptees: "The results of our longitudinal studies indicate that the long-term prognosis for adopted children is in no way worse than for children in the general population, provided that the adoptive home is well prepared for the task of rearing a nonbiological child. The study at 11 years admittedly indicated an increased frequency of nervous disturbances and maladjustment. This was, however, largely overcome in the subsequent follow-up studies."[2]

A minority of adoptees do want to search out their biological family, and this may well be a compelling case for open adoption, in which the mature child gains eventual access to records identifying the relinquishing parents. The Adoptees' Liberty Movement, formed in 1971, helps adoptees and birth parents to find each other and emphasizes that an adoptee should have access to adoption records, including the identity of his or her biological parents. But these complex and serious issues, while sometimes painful, do not negate the fundamental good of adoption: the adoptee at least has a life to live. It is wrong to misrepresent the incidence of usually quite temporary maladjustment of adoptees. The best current empirical evidence indicates that adoptees live good and productive lives, although their experience is unique.

Adoption was practiced in the Greek states and in Rome, among the Teutonic aristocracies and the Slavonic Russians and Poles. It was contained in the earliest codes of law, including that of Hammurabi.[3] It reached its widest acceptance in Rome. Unlike most of Europe, the English did not follow Roman precedent because of "an inordinately high regard for blood lineage and therefore the practice of adoption never acquired a foothold there."[4] Adoption in the Roman sense was made legally possible in England only in 1926, with the Adoption of Children Act. The United States, under the influence of English common law, did not develop adoption laws until the 1850s, when Spanish and French law began to have an effect on American society. We have had to struggle very hard, historically speaking, to bring adoption into our society, and even now the good that adoption can accomplish as an alternative to abortion or irresponsible instances of single parenthood is imperiled by the lack of moral support for relinquishing an infant. Yet, as Jeffrey Blustein has argued, the giving of children to others is *not* an unusual practice, and adoptive parents can do as well or better than biological ones in rearing a child.[5]

A VOLUNTARIST FRAMEWORK

Draconian approaches to adoption should be categorically rejected because of the grief that would result for the birth mother. In an important autobiographical study heralded as pivotal to understanding the birth mother's experience under coercive circumstances, Carol Schaeffer describes her dilemmas as a nineteen-year-old college freshman in 1965.[6] Pregnant, her boyfriend's family opposed marriage, she eventually signed papers for adoption, and the baby was taken away. But this was not authentically her desire, and she grieved. The grief remained, and she prayed daily for her son. When he reached eighteen years of age, she set out to find him. Against all odds, including denial of access to adoption records, she found her son after a two-year quest. The reunion was gratifying for both mother and son, and the adoptive parents were highly receptive. Schaeffer's criticism is *not* of relinquishing an infant per se, but of doing so less than wholeheartedly because of coercion.

The value of autonomy is essential to the cause of adoption. The feminist Barbara Katz Rothman writes, "For every baby taken in, there is a baby given up."[7] Months of physical intimacy in pregnancy, Rothman continues, cannot be dismissed—there is a loss. Yet, from the rich experiential sources she cites, it is clear that women who relinquish an infant freely and altruistically do not suffer unbearably from their grief. Rothman quotes a poem, written by a birth mother content with relinquishment:

> *I loved you and still do*
> *But I can't let that love in my life.*
> *I gave you life so your mother could love you.*
> *I signed the papers that said I was "Abandoning" you,*
> *But with love,*
> *With the knowledge that a family waited for you,*
> *Waited with joyous outstretched arms.*
> *I've seen the joy of families with special babies*
> *Like you.*
> *It is matchless.*
> *I've no regrets.*[8]

This poem is contrasted with one by Helen Garcia, who described her experience of relinquishment under social pressure as "Doin Time":

> *In the night we feel*
> *Sorrow, the twisting, churning*
> *Of nothingness*[9]

Rothman interprets this disparity of experience thus: "The birth mother without regrets may express and come to terms with her grief. The loss is there, but she can live with it, take satisfaction in the joy she created, the life she created and gave away."[10] But the birth mother with regrets cannot overcome her grief and is "Doin Time."

Rothman argues against pressure and forced choice. "It is not this choice that leads to the regret," she adds, "but the *force.*" Birth mothers who relinquish infants with a "deep sense of the rightness of what they are doing" can feel good about themselves, about the generosity of their acts.[11]

This newly emergent literature in women's studies about the experience of relinquishing an infant confirms the importance of its being voluntary and unpressured. The writings offer a corrective to coercive suggestions, the most notable being that of Raymond M. Herbenick. He argues that any woman who would make a voluntary decision to abort is guilty of abandonment in utero. Such abandonment justifies state custody of the infant for its own good and for "legitimate redistributive interests on behalf of minorities denied the equal opportunity of parenthood" because of infertility.[12] According to Herbenick, "a parent in an elective abortion and abandonment" decision should be required to carry the fetus to term in order to provide others with fair equality of parental opportunity. Needless to say, such an approach is disrespectful of autonomy and would be deeply offensive to women.

A voluntarist approach is taken in the important article on adoption dealing with clinical medical ethics, "A Physician's Guide to Adoption." The article suggests that physicians caring for women with unwanted pregnancies should explore nonjudgmentally the three options of abortion, adoption, and raising their children. The authors contend that because placing an infant for adoption is currently out of vogue, physicians are sometimes reluctant to open the subject for fear of alienating patients. Moreover, because "adoption is almost universally rejected by black women with unintended pregnancies, this option may be ignored inappropriately in the usual prenatal counseling of black women."[13] Physicians and other health care professionals, it is argued, need not be apologetic about addressing adoption in a knowledgeable manner and ought to have essential resources on hand. The article is especially critical of physicians who treat infertility but are (allegedly) unwilling to acknowledge failure and to broach the subject of adoption.

Those who defend adoption as a valid alternative suggest ways to alleviate the pain of relinquishing an infant. One partial solution is more "perceptive health care" for the relinquishing mother. In the hospital environment, a value-neutral terminology may be helpful. "Put up for adoption," "real" or "natural" parent, and so forth are terms to be avoided." "Placing a baby for adoption" is preferable to "giving up a baby." Since relinquishing one's infant can be like "experiencing a perinatal death," a supportive environment is essential.[14] Also, the birth mother should know that she will have access to nonidentifying information about her child as he or she grows up. Women who are considering placing a child should be cared for sensitively, and even more so immediately after the child has been given to its caring adoptive parents.

Even in the most sensitive of circumstances, it is safe to assume that relinquishing an infant is emotionally difficult, if not traumatic. This is why in a society that no longer views single parenthood with shame, and in which abortion is available on demand, placing a child for adoption is a hard sell. Nevertheless, giving something as precious as one's infant to others, while difficult, can be lauded as a beneficent act, one that makes possible the experience of parenthood for others.

A woman relinquishing her child should know that it is in good hands, and that she has provided adoptive parents with a remarkable opportunity. In modern times, many infertile couples take advantage of reproductive technologies. But more often than not, these technologies fail. By most estimates, the failure rate is about 80 percent for couples who attempt in vitro techniques multiple times. Unfortunately, some fertility clinics have exaggerated the success rate. For those who are unable to conceive their own child, adoption affords an opportunity for moral growth in the context of steadfast commitment and responsibility; it requires a level of self-transcendence or altruism that morally enriches parents; it demands that one live at least as much for the child as for oneself, and sometimes more so. Those who want to become parents but are frustrated by infertility or some other obstacle deserve to have this desire met insofar as efforts to encourage voluntary relinquishment permit.

An activist voluntarism is suggested by Cynthia B. Martin, a noted authority on adoption in America. "Adoption has no effective advocates," she writes, and adds, "Outreach programs and searches for potential biological parents to place children for adoption are unheard of. We do not recruit babies! I don't know why not." Martin argues that balanced pregnancy counseling is a deception because seldom are young women given the opportunity to explore equally all the possible alternatives. Most counseling agencies, she contends, simply do not mention adoption. Martin suggests a retrieval of adoption in pregnancy counseling: "With fewer babies available today than ever before, adoption is a viable, healthy alternative to unwanted pregnancy and needs to be promoted. It is time to try new, open, and different approaches to adoption. . . . It is time to make adoption a desirable, known alternative the pregnant woman might consider."[15]

Martin's allegations about the omission of mention of adoption in some settings may be true, but I have serious doubts that there are many women with unwanted pregnancies who are generally unaware of the adoption alternative. I do agree with Martin that more communication between prospective parents seeking a child and women with unwanted pregnancies is good, because surely those who desire an adoptive child have a story to tell that merits attentive listening and compassionate response. Perhaps the unhappily pregnant woman would consider placing her infant were she more aware of the current scarcity of children available for prospective parents. My sympathy lies with a suggestion made by Richard N. Levy: "Somehow a coalition should be able to develop of those who want but cannot bear and those who bear but do not want."[16] This sympathy need not be linked with an anti-choice position on abortion.

THE BESTOWAL OF PARENTAL LOVE

While I reject all coercive approaches to birth mothers, there is much to be said for providing couples with the opportunity of parenthood. The study of love in philosophical thought has been largely inattentive to the special affection that most parents have toward their children. This love was called *storge* by the Greeks, referring to affection generally but more especially to that of parents for offspring. Parenting is an important opportunity for husband and wife to learn the art of loving. In *storge* much of the beneficence in our world is grounded; love learned within the crucible of the parent-child relation can expand to encompass others, albeit stripped of any parentalist inequalities, as a pebble cast into water creates ripples that travel outward. Genuine love of humanity often—but obviously not always—has its beginnings in learning to love persons closest to us and for whom we are most responsible. Although Judaism and Christianity are in many respects discontinuous, it is possible to speak of a Judeo-Christian tradition regarding the image of parental *storge* as following a pattern of divine creation. The Jewish *chesed*, or "steadfast love," is most frequently captured in the Hebrew Bible by the intimate familial love of parent for child. The late Protestant ethicist Paul Ramsey articulated the Christian continuation of such: "Of course, we cannot see into the mystery of how God's love created the world. . . . Nevertheless, we procreate new beings like ourselves in the midst of our love for one another, and in this there is a trace of the original mystery by which God created the world.[17] The steadfast love that was *storge* to the Greeks brings together parental creation and nurturing affections that Judeo-Christian thought elevates to the sanctity of divine image. A natural theology, presuming that something of the character of the creator can be gleaned from creation, must view man and woman bringing a child into the world amidst steadfast love as *in imagine Dei* (in the image of God). Saint Paul wrote that God's attributes "have been visible, ever since the world began, to the eye of reason, in the things he has made" (Romans 1:20), and according to Genesis 1:28, man and woman together are in the image of God, who implicitly then is a being of parental love in its fullest expression.

The feminist theologian Sally McFague writes of God as mother-father-parental love, and comments, "Parental love is the most powerful and intimate experience we have of giving love to those whose return is not calculated (though a return is appreciated)." The moral ideal she suggests is to "see ourselves as universal parents, as profoundly desiring not our own lives to go on forever but the lives of others to come into being." Our essential task is to "universalize parenthood."[18] She views parenthood as an opportunity for moral growth in the parent.

Given the importance attached to the bestowal of parental love with respect to virtue and responsibility, those who desire it but cannot biologically create it deserve moral attention. They have no "right" to a child, and the woman with an unwanted pregnancy has no enforceable duty to relinquish her infant. In the sphere of charity and compassion, however, placing an infant in the hands of competent and desiring adoptive parents is pure gain for them. I would have no objection to a couple's conceiving a child (absent any financial incentives) for the specific purpose of relinquishing it to a childless couple, as has been the general practice for centuries in Asia, generally within a clan circle.

ABORTION TRAUMA

Advocates of adoption have made exaggerated claims that women who undergo abortions inevitably suffer psychological damages, and so relinquishing an infant is the less traumatic option and therefore more morally acceptable. Some have argued that there is a measurable phenomenon called "postabortion syndrome" (PAS). But PAS is an ideological fabrication and one that confuses psychological disease with the experience of compunction. All that can and need be said is that some women have reported a sense of moral guilt in the wake of abortion, usually some years after the event. This hardly makes a strong case for carrying a fetus to term and relinquishing it to others.

On the question of abortion trauma, Dr. C. Everett Koop, then surgeon general of the United States, wrote a controversial letter to Ronald Reagan, then president, in which he claimed that after extensive review of the available social-scientific studies, it was impossible to conclude that women were harmed by abortions. Specifically, wrote Koop, "scientific studies do not provide conclusive data about the effects of abortion on women."[19] Physical harms such as infertility, premature birth, and miscarriage are difficult to attribute to previous abortions, and psychological effects such as depression cannot be clearly established, he argued. Moreover, conclusive data would require an extended five-year study following thousands of women from before they conceived. The authors of a study published in 1989 suggest that "abortion is not experienced as particularly traumatic by the majority of women postabortion," and that those who do suffer psychological trauma either blame the pregnancy on another person or on their own character.[20] The results of this study, however, are based only on follow-up testing of women three weeks after abortion.

Those who think that so-called PAS is a reality for some women argue that it surfaces between five and seven years after abortion and so a three-week study is too short. They also contend that many women are pleased with the decision to abort insofar as it affects their current circumstances, repressing the trauma that might surface much later at various levels of intensity.

Another study, based on a two-year assessment of 360 teenage black women, concludes that those who abort are free from trauma. The authors acknowledge, however, that "only a longitudinal study of a randomly selected group of young women that begins long before their exposure to abortion could permit the performance of an accurate psychological appraisal, uncontaminated by the effects of a suspected pregnancy."[21] Critics point out that two years is still too short a time period and that support groups for women with PAS exist in virtually every region of the country.[22]

Although these studies can be criticized, they do point out that post-abortion trauma is difficult, if not impossible, to demonstrate empirically, as Koop suggested. Even in a lengthier study over a decade, generalizations from individual experiences of abortion would be exceedingly difficult to make because of the variables involved. Is a middle-aged woman with children likely to suffer in conscience whereas a younger woman with no children will not? Would a woman who aborts while young and then is unable to conceive a desired child later in life be likely to attribute her current suffering to a past abortion? How much do shifting religious and moral worldviews affect the way in which women later reinterpret their abortion? It may be impossible to make any accurate measurement of grief due to abortion because there are so many variables.

Some interesting anecdotal material suggests that abortion can leave at least some woman with a disturbing burden of guilt. Linda Bird Franke describes the case of "Jane Doe," thirty-eight years old in 1973, the year of her abortion. The mother of three children already, Jane and her husband thought that a fourth child would be overburdening. But Jane did not anticipate the guilt that followed years after her abortion: "And it certainly does make more sense not to be having a baby right now—we say that to each other all the time. But I have this little ghost now. A very little ghost that only appears when I'm seeing something beautiful, like the full moon on the ocean last weekend. And the baby waves at me. And I wave at the baby. 'Of course, we have room,' I cry to the ghost. 'Of course we do.'"[23] These are the words of an individual woman, living with considerable guilt.

It cannot be assumed that such anxiety is typical of women who have had abortions. Many may acknowledge a sense of moral guilt, but given similar circumstances they would still make the same choice. Still, their stories suggest that abortion is at least not morally inconsequential, and presumably few women who choose abortion are unaware of this.

If there is a locus classicus on this matter, it would be the book *Surfacing*, by the Canadian feminist Margaret Atwood. The protagonist in *Surfacing* speaks for Atwood, who felt deep remorse after having an abortion. Here are some of her retrospective thoughts and experiences:

> It was there when I woke up, suspended in the air above me like a chalice, an evil grail and I thought, Whatever it is, part of myself or a separate creature, I killed it. It wasn't a child but it could have been one, I didn't allow it.[24]

> It was real enough, it was enough reality for ever. I couldn't accept it, that mutilation, ruin I'd made, I needed a different version.[25]

> Since then I'd carried that death around inside me, layering it over, a cyst, a tumor, black pearl.[26]

> He trembles and then I can feel my lost child surfacing within me, forgiving me, rising from the lake where it has been prisoned for so long, its eyes and teeth phosphorescent; the two halves clasp, interlocking like fingers, it buds, it sends out fronds.[27]

These passages are powerful because they emerge from the author's personal experience and enable us to have some sense of Atwood's strained conscience.

But as Carol P. Christ points out, the protagonist in *Surfacing* suffered remorse largely because she allowed her lover to choose abortion for her, "and because she did not allow herself to feel the sense of loss that will naturally be felt when a life is taken."[28] The protagonist's resentment against those who imposed a decision on her clearly underlies her guilt.

Were abortion trauma ever demonstrated, this trauma would have to be balanced with the trauma of going through with an unwanted pregnancy, or with the emotional difficulties of placing an infant for adoption. It is the latter that concerns us here, for many women find it terribly difficult to relinquish their children. These women may themselves acknowledge that abortion is not a matter of little consequence, but they will add that it appears less traumatic than not knowing or seeing their children. Indeed, this seems to have been the view of "Jane Roe," of *Roe vs. Wade*, who could not accept relinquishing a second infant.

In summary, the recovery of more positive attitudes among pregnant women toward placing an infant for adoption will not benefit from empirically suspect indictments of abortion respecting its supposed negative consequences for women. This recovery, if it is to proceed at all, must be focused on the moral meaning of relinquishing an infant to those who desire to experience parenthood and to bestow parental love. The appeal must be to the virtue of beneficence, not to abortion traumas.

AN APPEAL FOR BENEFICENCE

The feminist Rosalind Hursthouse underscores an important reason why many women prefer abortion to relinquishing an infant:

> Indeed, it seems that many women who opt for abortion rather than pregnancy followed by adoption, despite believing that abortion is wrong, do so because they cannot contemplate the idea without pain. Some say that if they had the baby they know they could not bring themselves to have it adopted, so their choice has to lie between abortion and having a child that they bring up. Others say that if they had the baby and had it adopted they would always worry about how it was getting on, and what had become of it.[29]

Although Hursthouse relies on anecdotal evidence, it is reasonable to acknowledge that, for some women, the emotional strain from the anticipation of never seeing their child again discourages the choice for adoption.

Placing an infant for adoption is not entirely disanalogous to surrogate mothering, and it is well known that sometimes the birth mother finds parting with the infant to be difficult if not impossible. Elizabeth S. Anderson writes of the grief such relinquishment can entail: "The treatment and interpretation of surrogate mothers' grief raises the deepest problems of degradation. Most surrogate mothers experience grief upon giving up their children—in 10 percent of cases, seriously enough to require therapy."[30]

Mary Beth Whitehead finally could not bear the torment of leaving her biological child with the Sternses, despite having signed a surrogacy contract. Although there are important discontinuities between adoption and surrogacy, the controversy over the latter does drive home the anguish some women experience in relinquishing a child.

Certainly the wider historical tradition of Western ethical thought is not unsympathetic with the view that relinquishment is "unnatural." Ramsey, as referred to above, writes that in procreating, human beings must nurture their children, for in this "is a trace of the original mystery by which God created the world." Here Protestantism echoes a longstanding emphasis in the medieval Catholic ethics of natural law. Thomas Aquinas borrowed from the third-century Roman jurist Ulpian in claiming that human beings should live according to nature as do the animals, rearing the children they bring into the world. Charles J. McFadden, S.J., summed up the Catholic norm as follows: "In this respect, man can learn much from the animals in lower creation. Natural instinct compels the beast to exhibit a tender care and self-sacrificing solicitude for its young."[31] Begetting, loving, and rearing ordinarily should go hand in hand. Thus, those women who feel that they could not bear to give up a child, and that to do so would be unnatural, should not be dismissed as morally solipsistic and faddish. Instead, their reluctance should be taken most seriously and as embedded in the wider tradition.

In a study by the Guttmacher Institute, based on data from 1985, it is estimated that there are about 3 million unintended pregnancies annually in the United States. Of 1.5 million babies born following such pregnancies, only about 2 percent are placed for adoption. The large majority of women who do not abort decide to keep their babies, viewing relinquishment as "unnatural." Up to the early 1970s it was generally understood that an infant born out of wedlock would be adopted; this is obviously no longer the case. According to Elizabeth S. Cole, director of the Permanent

Family for Children Project of the Child Welfare League of America, adoption, once thought to be the ideal solution to pregnancy when marriage for the parents was not possible, is now frowned on by a generation of young women: "At a recent conference of pregnancy counsellors, there was a great deal of discussion concerning the fact that many pregnant teenagers are pressured by their peers not to give up their child, as the giving is 'unnatural.'"[32] It is thus well documented that many pregnant women nowadays reject adoption. Times have changed, due in part to the powerful cultural consequences of abortion on demand and to nontraditional views of the family. The preferred, more "natural" solutions to an unwanted pregnancy are abortion, or else the raising of children without fathers. For prospective adoptive couples, this cultural transition is not good.

A CULTURAL POSSIBILITY?

As has already been stated, adoption has a long historical legacy in most societies. We cannot easily reconstruct the cultural, moral, and institutional supports necessary for the restoration of the practice of relinquishing an infant to the care of others, but reflection on an earlier era shows that such construction is not impossible. The development of a coalition between those who want but cannot bear and those who bear but do not want is certainly a possibility. Just what shape this coalition would take I do not venture to suggest, although the funding of homes for unwed pregnant women and an educational outreach emphasizing the needs of childless couples would be reasonable options.

History is instructive with respect to cultural possibilities that are sometimes forgotten. In a remarkable survey of the Western practice of adoption through the Renaissance, the historian John Eastburn Boswell concludes, "Society relied on the kindness of strangers to protect its extra children, a kindness much admired and prominent in the public consciousness." Boswell contends that Europe relied on a "panoply of formal and informal arrangements" for giving children away. The chief motive for abandonment was poverty, "and the church met the needs of poor parents by providing a safe location to leave children and a system for placing them."[33] Abandonment was a form of exposition—not exposure—

intended to remove a child "from the family's responsibility, not from life."[34] Many children were adopted as free sons and daughters by parents who were either childless or had lost their own children. Biological parents viewed their offerings as "laudable," rather than "morally neutral." This was a way of "returning fruits to the Lord," and "in Christian society the giving up of a child for a greater good could hardly have had greater subliminal religious significance."[35]

Boswell acknowledges that when a child was placed in the hands of others, the "cost to the parents was the emotional sacrifice."[36] The ideal of sacrificial love for others was a profound norm in medieval Europe, best symbolized by the pelican plucking its chest veins in order to provide blood for its offspring's sustenance. Out of self-denying love a parent could do what was necessary for the well-being of an infant, and for those who were childless. Self-sacrifice was a high ideal that encouraged couples to relinquish their children as an act of beneficence for both the children relinquished and for those who received them. A willingness to endure emotional pain when necessary for the good of an infant one loves, an "ideal of nonbiological, fostering love,"[37] a nonproprietary attitude toward one's children, a compassion for those who are without children of their own, and most of all the "kindness of strangers" made relinquishing an infant a morally compelling act.

A culture of adoption is not widely recoverable, since now no shame is associated with single parenting (it is chic in some circles), and abortion is both safe and perfectly routine. What recovery might be made must be predicated on compassion for those who would adopt but can find no reasonably healthy infants available. A certain moral idealism is needed.

A FREE OPTION

Those who currently defend adoption on moral grounds, particularly Herbenick and James T. Burtchaell, view it as the necessary and imposed alternative to abortion.[38] In contrast, I prefer to see adoption as one of the points of common ground between those who are pro-life, pro-choice, or both. Women bearing unwanted infants, childless couples wanting to raise a son or daughter, pro-choice advocates, pro-life advocates, and adoptees themselves could work together to make adoption a significant option fairly presented and defended.

What might be done? Environments could be created in which pregnant women would be supported both financially and emotionally in order to give birth and relinquish their infants in a sensitive environment. Counseling should be offered so that women who relinquish a child can deal creatively with ambivalence, and so that the choice to relinquish can be judged authentic and genuinely free. Women should *never* relinquish infants unwillingly. They should have the opportunity to meet with childless couples who desire to have a child. The possibilities for collaboration that would benefit the pregnant woman, the unborn, and the childless are myriad.

Family planning and pregnancy counselors should be as much a part of this adoption network as they are a part of the abortion network. They should not be directive, but neither should they, by omission, encourage abortion rather than adoption. (Whether this omission currently occurs is a matter of some controversy.) For an adoption coalition to succeed, it will take national commitment and philanthropic resolve.

NOTES

1. David M. Brodzinsky, "A Stress and Coping Model of Adoption Adjustment," in David M. Brodzinsky and Marshall D. Schechter, eds., *The Psychology of Adoption* (New York: Oxford University Press, 1990), p. 23.

2. Michael Bohman and Søren Sigvardsson, "Outcome in Adoption: Lessons from Longitudinal Studies," in Brodzinsky and Schechter, *The Psychology of Adoption*, p. 104.

3. Irving J. Stone, *The Law of Adoption and Surrogate Parenting* (New York: Oceana Publications, 1988), p. 7.

4. Ibid., p. 8.

5. Jeffrey Blustein, *Parents and Children: The Ethics of the Family* (New York: Oxford University Press, 1982).

6. Carol Schaeffer, *The Other Mother: A Woman's Love for the Child She Gave Up for Adoption* (New York: Soho Press, 1991).

7. Barbara Katz Rothman, *Recreating Motherhood: Ideology and Technology in a Patriarchal Society* (New York: W. W. Norton, 1989), p. 126.

8. Ibid., p. 128.

9. Ibid., p. 129.

10. Ibid.

11. Ibid., p. 130.

12. Raymond M. Herbenick, "Remarks on Abortion, Abandonment, and Adoption Opportunities," in Onora O'Neill and William Ruddick, eds., *Having Children: Philosophical and Legal Reflections on Parenthood* (New York: Oxford University Press, 1979), p. 55.

13. Andrew M. Kaunitz, David A. Grimes, and Karen K. Koppel, "A Physician's Guide to Adoption," *Journal of the American Medical Association* 258 (1987): 3538.

14. Ibid., p. 3539.

15. Cynthia D. Martin, *Beating the Adoption Game* (New York: Harcourt Brace Jovanovich, 1988), pp. 19–20, 22.

16. Richard N. Levy, "Abortion and Its Alternatives," *Sh'ma: A Journal of Jewish Responsibility* 8, no. 144 (1977): 214.

17. Paul Ramsey, *Fabricated Man: The Ethics of Genetic Control* (New Haven: Yale University Press, 1970), p. 38.

18. Sally McFague, *Models of God: Theology for an Ecological Nuclear Age* (Philadelphia: Fortress Press, 1987), pp. 103, 119, 121.

19. M. Tolchin, "Koop's Stand on Abortion's Effect Surprises Friends and Foes Alike," *New York Times,* 11 January 1989, p. A11.

20. Pallas Mueller and Brenda Major, "Self-Blame, Self-Efficacy, and Adjustment to Abortion," *Journal of Personality and Social Psychology* 57, no. 6 (1989): 1059.

21. Laurie Schwab Zabin, Marilyn B. Hirsh, and Mark R. Emerson, "When Urban Adolescents Choose Abortion: Effects on Education, Psychological Status, and Subsequent Pregnancy," *Family Planning Perspectives* 21, no. 6 (1989): 248.

22. Chris Raymond, "Studies of Abortion's Emotional Effects Renew Controversial Scholarly Debate," *Chronicle of Higher Education,* 7 February 1990, 6.

23. Linda Bird Franke, *The Ambivalence of Abortion* (New York: Random House, 1978), p. 84.

24. Margaret Atwood, *Surfacing* (New York: Fawcett Crest, 1972), pp. 167–168.

25. Ibid., p. 168.

26. Ibid., p. 170.

27. Ibid., p. 193.

28. Carol P. Christ, *Diving Deep and Surfacing: Women Writers on Spiritual Quest* (Boston: Beacon Press, 1980), p. 98.

29. Rosalind Hursthouse, *Beginning Lives* (Oxford: Basil Blackwell, 1987), pp. 210–211.

30. Elizabeth S. Anderson, "Is Women's Labor a Commodity?" *Philosophy and Public Affairs* 19, no. 1 (1990): 84.

31. Charles J. McFadden, *Medical Ethics* (Philadelphia: F. A. Davis, 1956), p. 53.

32. Elizabeth S. Cole, "Societal Influence on Adoption Practices," in Paul Sachdev, ed., *Adoption: Current Issues and Trends* (Toronto: Butterworths, 1984), p. 18.

33. John Eastborn Boswell, *The Kindness of Strangers: The Abandonment of Children in Western Europe from Late Antiquity to the Renaissance* (New York: Pantheon, 1988), pp. 256, 433.

34. John Eastburn Boswell, "Expositio and *Oblatio:* The Abandonment of Children and the Ancient and Medieval Family," *American Historical Review* 89, no. 1 (1984): 13.

35. Ibid., p. 241.

36. Ibid., p. 240.

37. Ibid., p. 239.

38. James T. Burtchaell, *Rachael Weeping: The Case against Abortion* (San Francisco: Harper and Row, 1984).

3

Adolescents in Time of AIDS: Values and Preventive Education

There are few areas of public health more controversial than the prevention of acquired immunodeficiency syndrome, or AIDS, since differences in values often result in acrimonious debate. I focus on AIDS prevention and adolescents because they are at risk in a period of their lives when concern with mortality is often slight. There are two basic strategies that are used in the education of adolescents on prevention of AIDS. The first is morally directive, stressing the postponement of sexual involvement and the value of long-term mutual fidelity between people who are free of sexually transmitted disease. The second is morally nondirective and technological, stressing the protective benefits of latex barriers. I call the second solution "technofix." Technofix is unreliable. As Nicholas Freudenberg writes in a report published under the imprimatur of the American Public Health Association, "Studies of contraceptive effectiveness show that condoms fail to prevent pregnancy for at least one couple out of ten who rely on the method for a year. Many studies show even higher failure rate. It is likely that HIV [human immunodeficiency virus] transmission occurs more readily than conception." I agree with his conclusion that responsible AIDS educators must talk "positively and accurately" about condoms but "without giving learners a false sense of security."[1]

Because technofix is insecure, I consider it imperative to begin education with frank discussion of what love really is and of uncommitted sex as a false substitute for real love. On some existential level, I think, most people understand this falseness, so intelligent conversation is possible regardless of religious background or the lack thereof. (For purposes of this discussion, HIV transmission by way of needles is set aside.)

There is hard debate between those who would emphasize moral directiveness and those who stress the allegedly more "realistic" technofix. For example, a majority of four on the New York City Board of Education voted in May 1992 for an AIDS prevention curriculum that devotes substantially more time and attention to postponement than to other forms of prevention. An angry outburst followed from some parents, students, and teachers, and from the schools chancellor. But as one reporter indicated, there were also students claiming that "the ideal of sexual abstinence has not been given enough of a chance" and that "the possibilities of condom failure" are ignored.[2]

Legitimate questions of sexual morality should not be dismissed as the "moralistic" importing of moral concerns where they have no place, or as merely "political." On the contrary, it would be irresponsible not to consider the moral question. A nineteen-year-old woman infected by HIV reports that her doctor recommended she contact anyone she had been sexually active with during the previous year. "It was easy for me to list the guys I had slept with," she says, "but when I counted 24, I was like, gosh!"[3]

An adequate AIDS-preventive education for adolescents must make the postponement of sexual intimacy a part of its content. The approach I suggest includes four components: presentation of the facts of HIV infection during adolescence; discussion of ethics, sex, and love; development of refusal skills taught through role-playing techniques; and presentation for those who wish to hear it on the clear benefits of condom usage and the reality of failure rates.

Before describing the content of this four-part approach, I hasten to point out that the values of postponement and mutual fidelity have been a large part of the preventive response to AIDS among homosexuals and adult heterosexuals. It is therefore unreasonable that these values are not welcomed by some educators as fit possibilities for adolescents. Steven Seidman has documented the shift from indiscriminate sex and "hedonistic preoccupations of gay men to a new ethic of sexual and social responsibility."[4] The free-wheeling promiscuous lifestyle of sexual libertarians has been significantly replaced by fidelity or abstinence. Among heterosexuals disenchanted with the sexual revolution and concerned with their physical and emotional health, a powerful movement to rediscover the nonsexual has been under way since about 1980, when Gabrielle Brown's *The New Celibacy* was first published. In a later edition, Brown points out that the new celibacy is not simply due to fear of AIDS and other sexually transmitted diseases but to support for the "decasualization of sex." She is critical of "an overenriched conception of sexual behavior," whereby "people end up thinking they are more sexual than they really are. And they feel they should live up to a false picture of sexuality that has been created as a standard."[5]

THE FACTS OF AIDS AND THE ADOLESCENT

In 1992, William Roper, a public health specialist and the director of the national Centers for Disease Control and Prevention (CDC), issued a report entitled "U.S. Youth Risk Behavior Survey, 1990," indicating that American high school students were playing "Russian roulette" with AIDS. The report, which was the culmination of a CDC study of 11,631 high school students throughout the United States, revealed that 54.2 percent of high school students had had sexual intercourse (60.8 percent male, 48 percent female), compared with 29 percent in 1970, and 29 percent of high school seniors had had four or more sexual partners. In addition to indicating the results of this study, the report also points out that more than 800 people between the ages of thirteen and nineteen and 8,402 between the ages of twenty and twenty-four had been diagnosed as having AIDS (since it can take ten or more years for HIV infection to become full-fledged AIDS, these numbers indicate widespread adolescent HIV infection); many people who manifest AIDS in their twenties contracted it in adolescence; in the last two years, AIDS cases among those between thirteen and twenty-four years have increased 77 percent.[6] In response to this peril, the CDC recommends that "education programs should provide adolescents with the knowledge, attitudes, and skills they need to refrain from sexual intercourse. For adolescents who are unwilling to refrain from sexual intercourse, programs should help to increase the use of contraception and condoms." One CDC goal is to see a reduction of 15 percent in the number of adolescents who are sexually active by age fifteen and a reduction of 40 percent in those active by age seventeen. With a concerted effort these goals are deemed realistic.

Educational efforts are more successful if adolescents with HIV or AIDS speak from their experience, thereby creating an emotional event in the lives of young listeners. In addition to personalizing the epidemic, this approach demonstrates how an infected individual can be virtually unidentifiable.[7]

ETHICS, SEX, AND LOVE

But what should the first educational point be? In my view, it should be that our culture desperately needs to recover the link between sex and love, and the insight that love, to be worthy of the word, does not require sexual expression. Love manifests in a deep caring for the welfare of the other; it is a rejection of the self-centered tendency and a transfer of interests to another for his or her own sake. Myriad partial definitions can be combined to suggest that love includes joy, compassion, commitment, and respect: love rejoices in the health, existence, growth, and presence of the other; love never harms; love responds to the suffering of the other; love is committed and patient; love honors the other's freedom, integrity, and individuality, including the freedom to refuse sexual intimacy. Love generally exists without any sexual expression, for example, in parental love, love of children for parents, friendship, or compassion for the suffering. Even in married love, a person may suffer a physical condition that precludes sex, but love can and should continue on. An especially vile violation of love occurs when someone knowingly transmits HIV to another.

One necessary response to AIDS lies in a moral rejection of the assumption that happiness is achieved as a matter of course through liberation from the boundary of love and commitment within the context of mutual and creative fidelity. Few would deny that sexual license is responsible for vast harms. As the psychiatrist Willard Gaylin states, "the only empirical results of that illegitimate offspring of Freudian philosophy, the sexual revolution, seem to be the spread of two sexually transmitted diseases, genital herpes and AIDS; an extraordinary rise in the incidence of cancer of the cervix; and a disastrous epidemic of teenage pregnancies."[8]

In the final analysis, death from AIDS is largely preventable through sexual morality.

From a public health perspective, the record of the sexual revolution is disastrous. The rise in primary- and secondary-stage syphilis and chlamydia is significant. Human papillomavirus, related to 80 percent of all cervical cancers, is estimated to be carried by between 10 and 30 percent of all Americans. Tragically, the highest incidence of cervical cancer is among those between the ages of nineteen and thirty. With a gap of seven to ten years between precancerous cellular changes and the onset of cancer, this age group suffers the results of carelessness during adolescence.

Roper believes that we must apply antismoking fervor to high-risk sexual behavior among teens, citing studies indicating that 40 percent of students at the University of California at Berkeley have had a sexually transmitted disease.[9] What is required is a revolt against sex outside of monogamous and mutually faithful relationships, and against the assumption that there is no moral difference between sex and the contraction of a leg muscle or eating junk food. Until we address these deeper concerns, our children will increasingly confront early death.

Blame rests with parents, churches, teachers, media, and all people or institutions failing to enter fully into discussion not only about the connection between sex and deadly disease but about the loss of the higher meanings of love that should direct and inform sexual intimacy. Sexual intimacy, which manifests a rich and beautiful significance when sought within the proper hierarchy of values, within the permanent commitment to the full well-being of the beloved, is debased by a culture gone awry. We must not be afraid to speak this truth and to exemplify it in our own behavior.

Teachers of ethics and moral philosophy have much to say about social ethics, but fewer enter the domain of sexual ethics. Students read Kant's theories, but seldom are they asked to consider his comments on sex. Yet Kant strongly articulated that sexual desire often reduces its objects to mere means. He commented at length on how morally problematic the "appetite for another human being" can be, adding that "there is no way in which a human being can be made an object of indulgence for another except through sexual impulse." It is a simple fact, Kant contends, that through sexual appetite one human being often plunges another into "the depths of misery," casting him or her aside "as one casts away a lemon which has been sucked dry."[10] The analogy is powerful and fitting.

A final result of the sexual revolution is emotional despair and a sense of meaninglessness. Paul R. Fleischman, a psychiatrist and theologian, writes that if sexual repression dominated the psychological landscape in Freud's Vienna, the current problem is quite the reverse: "Among the hurt and pained in need of help, who may suffer from broken marriages, fluctuating or fallen self-esteem, obsessive constrictions, panicky attachments to parents, bewildering isolation, uncontrolled rages, and haunting depressions, the common denominator is an inability to transcend themselves with care and delight, to reach over and touch another heart." Fleischman's patients report that they suffer emotionally because they have assumed that genuine love requires sexual intimacy. They then pursue such relations, even when inappropriate, and suffer the consequences. Their experience may be summed up thus: "The binding together, the touch of person to person, is sought concretely, rather than spiritually, and dyadically rather than communally. The substitution of sexuality for religious life constitutes one of the most prominent and pervasive elements of cultural pathology that a psychotherapist encounters."[11] Many people seek to touch physically for the sake of sexual intimacy alone, failing to see physical touch as at all expressive of a deeper spiritual meaning. They make sexual intimacy rather than nonphysical values the center of their lives.

Pride, the desire to dominate others, self-assertion, and egocentrism—all radically inconsistent with love—animate the sexual preoccupations that destroy love. Our culture of flight from restraint disguises these grim realities in order to reject nonsexualized values in our relations with others. Sin has been redefined by popular culture as *not* expressing libido, and restraint is construed as negative and repressive. The possibility of arguing for sexual restraint without diminishing the glory of the erotic is not contemplated.

Modern innovations have audaciously shaped the contemporary world in a way that has made us antagonistic to the restraints that make moral and spiritual development possible. It is not barbarous superstition to suggest that the body should be honored as the seat of a higher principle.

Twenty years ago the psychiatrist Rollo May warned eloquently about the changing American morality. He wrote, "The Victorian nice man or woman was guilty if he or she did experience sex; now we are guilty if we *don't.*" May continues, "What we did not see in our short-sighted liberalism in sex was that throwing the individual into an unbounded and empty sea of free choice does not in itself give freedom, but is more apt to cause inner conflict."[12] He was concerned that a culture was emerging in which all love to be worthy of the word would require sexual expression and in which friendship and compassionate self-sacrifice would be displaced by "having sex." May was concerned with psychological harms. Now there is the added prognosis of death. The reality of AIDS should press us to educate the young about the sanctity of the body, about ways to resist the culturally enforced tyranny of oversexualization, and about the liberation in loving one another as friends. We can thus save young lives, and that is surely a common goal.

REFUSAL SKILLS

Knowing about the reality of AIDS as a risk, and about the spiritual and physical destruction of promiscuity, adolescents can begin to learn refusal skills through role playing. Role playing in which students act out roles in small skits they have written themselves tends to be effective. Students must learn that their task is to live meaningful, healthy, and happy lives, which probably will require them to tell someone kindly but firmly, "I do not yet desire or feel ready for sexual intimacy."

Attitudes favorable to postponement of sexual experience and to responsible behavior can be created, allowing adolescents to resist peer pressure. Students ask these kinds of questions in developing refusal skills: Am I sure no one is pushing me into sexual intimacy? Am I pushing my partner? When the relationship breaks up, will I be glad I was sexually intimate with this person? Am I willing to risk pregnancy and future infertility? Can I handle having an abortion, being a single parent, of placing my child up for adoption? Will sexual intimacy really make me more popular, more mature, more desirable? Is delaying sex better in the long run? Is sex the basis and goal of a deep and lasting love? What kinds of abuse and manipulation can occur in sexual relationships? Is it right that our culture puts the foremost emphasis on sexual pleasure? Are there other forms of pleasure? Aren't decisions about sex among the most important ones a person ever makes? How does uncommitted sex violate true love? Are some things in life so important that they are worth waiting for?

On the simplest level, adolescents need to know how to say no. Lines like these surface in skits I have witnessed in church work with adolescents. "I like you, but I'm just not ready to be sexually intimate"; "I don't believe in sex before marriage, so I want to wait"; "I don't feel like sexual intimacy, and I don't need to give you a reason"; "Don't think that I owe you sex for taking me out to dinner. A simple thank you is sufficient!" Adolescents need to be prepared, if necessary, to find someone else whose thoughts on sex and love are closer to their own.

TECHNOFIX

Technofix is a preventive measure of great importance when postponement or fidelity is rejected. Adolescents who reject abstinence or fidelity should know among other things that latex condom failure is to be expected.

In a study published in the *Journal of the American Medical Association*, researchers point out that while undamaged latex condoms provide an effective barrier against "all known sexually transmissible agents, including HIV," the "significant slippage and breakage rates" in condom use indicate the need for a "backup virucidal barrier." The study concludes, "Condoms, even in combination with nonoxynol 9 [a spermaticide], probably will not provide absolute protection against HIV transmission. The best advice for persons with HIV infection is to abstain from vaginal or anorectal intercourse, and for those at risk of HIV infection, to engage in mutually monogamous relationships with a known HIV-negative partner."[13] (The efficacy of nonoxynol 9 in preventing HIV transmission is now doubted by researchers.)

In another study involving spousal transmission of HIV, one in ten HIV-infected individuals passed the virus on to their spouse despite using condoms.[14] This transmission rate of 10 percent occurs among spouses using careful condom techniques, so the rate is predictably higher among those who are less experienced. Moreover, "it appears difficult to achieve a high degree of condom use in most sexually active populations."[15]

The Board of Trustees of the American Medical Association makes a similar point: "A condom barrier offers some but not complete protection. Avoiding sexual contact and not sharing needles are the only sure protections."[16] Paul J. Feldblum and Judith A. Fortney state, "While the use of condoms or spermicides is unlikely to be harmful, there is potential harm if their use is substituted for abstinence, monogamy, or good judgment."[17] Vicki L. Seltzer, Jill Rabin, and Fred Benjamin write, "Obviously, the risk of sexually transmitted infection can be minimized optimally either with abstinence or by being sexually active only with a mutually faithful uninfected partner; this fact must be emphasized as well."[18]

Richard Gordon, the author of the most complete review of the literature on the efficacy of condoms in protecting against HIV transmission, concludes thus: "The effectiveness of condoms in preventing HIV transmission is much lower than their effectiveness in preventing pregnancy. This is because couples can conceive during only a small fraction of the menstrual cycle (the 'fertility window'). The condom failures that occur at other times do not increase pregnancy statistics. Thus the actual condom failure rate is much higher than pregnancy statistics indicate." Moreover, when condom failure rates are analyzed over extended periods of time, condoms "are inadequate from the point of view of the individual for lifetime protection from the AIDS epidemic, even with training and high motivation."[19] Again, about 10 percent of seronegative spouses convert to seropositive even when their infected partner uses condoms. Ezekiel J. Emanuel and Linda L. Emanuel of Harvard University, drawing on this 10 percent figure, reject the notion of the condom as safeguard: "Furthermore, it is ethically impermissible to use distorted slogans, partial information, and exaggerated claims; we cannot offer people false security in the hope of persuading them to act more prudently."[20]

Given the reality of condom failure, parents and others must begin to discuss the ethics of sex, and particularly the relationship between sex and love. In a powerful article appearing in the *New Zealand Medical Journal,* Neil D. Broom and Charles E. F. Rickett argue that an educational focus on condoms runs the risk of "abstracting the sexual area from the wider aspects of human personality." They continue persuasively: "In so doing there is a great danger of regarding sexually active or potentially active teenagers merely as copulating machines requiring only 'contraceptive services.'" The authors conclude that adolescents are "equally entitled to hear the opposite message—that there are positive physical and emotional advantages in adopting a philosophy of life that places the sexual experience within a committed and trusting relationship."[21]

FLIGHT FROM RESTRAINT

Our culture can be described as manifesting a mass flight from beneficial sexual restraint.[22] Although such flight is not new, its ubiquity in modernity may be. The toll of unrestraint on physical and emotional well-being has already been lamented. C. S. Lewis, for one, writing in the early 1950s, warned against the loss of any serious moral caution regarding sexual intimacy: "Poster after poster, film after film, novel after novel, associate the idea of sexual indulgence with the ideas of health, normality, youth, frankness, and good humour. Now this association is a lie." It is a lie, wrote Lewis, because sexual indulgence without commitment and steadfast love has always been associated with disease, deception, jealousies, and emotional pain. Lewis claimed that our society has lost sight of definitions of love that do not place sexual intimacy at their center, that it has illusory expectations of this intimacy, and the result is oppressive. He rejected the practice of sexual union when it is isolated "from all the other kinds of union which were intended to go along with it and make up the total union."[23]

The aim of restraint, as Kierkegaard argued, is the affirmation of good rather than the prohibition of evil. The task is to bring sexuality "under the qualification of the spirit (here lies all the moral problems of the erotic)."[24] The sexual revolution rejects all such qualification; its roots lie partially in nineteenth-century materialism and a view of the psychic life of human beings as the manifestation of processes in the physical organism. Eros, this materialism claimed, always aims at genital pleasure, the model of all human happiness; in the process Plato's "heavenly *eros*" lost its classical ground. The historians John D'Emilio and Estelle B. Freedman have shown that by the mid-1910s assumptions were commonplace that the sexual instinct demands constant expression, that restraint is harmful, and that gratification is a more worthy ideal than self-control. Thus, "the shift from a philosophy of continence to one that encouraged indulgence was but one aspect of a larger reorientation that was investing sexuality with a profoundly new importance."[25] All restraint was construed as negative and repressive. Arguing for sexual restraint without diminishing the glory of sexual Eros was now hardly tolerable.

Contemporary culture is preoccupied with sexual expression. This libertarianism severs relations between ethics, sexuality, spirituality, and artistic creativity. Our artists and writers rarely, if ever, adopt attitudes that recognize genuine love. This love does not require sexual expression and is therefore less marketable. Yet there is a need for artistic expression of the theme that love is at bottom spiritual and that the sexual expression of love is harmful and morally wrong outside of spiritual maturity and commitment.

The traditional notion of the sanctity of the human body has roots in Judaism, and Christianity's view of the body as God's temple is not without value. But we have lost this sense of the sanctity of the body. Our culture inculcates an overemphasis on sexual love. An ethical theory, although it may be a necessary condition of healing, cannot, all alone, reverse our flight. Metanoia, a basic transformation, is required, and that no theory can give. It is not barbarous superstition to suggest that the body should be honored as the seat of a higher principle, a notion that attracted Plato no less than Saint Paul.

In time of AIDS, no matter what someone's sexual orientation, technofix is helpful but ultimately inadequate. The AIDS epidemic can be virtually stopped when people decide to modify their behavior. It is not obvious that medical science will find a cure or an AIDS vaccine in the near future, if ever. A statement from the historian William H. McNeill is relevant: "Ingenuity, knowledge, and organization alter but cannot cancel humanity's vulnerability to invasion by parasitic forms of life."[26]

NOTES

1. Nicholas Freudenberg, *Preventing AIDS: A Guide to Effective Education for the Prevention of HIV Infection* (Washington, D.C.: American Public Health Association, 1989), p. 99.

2. Joseph Berger, "Where the Facts of AIDS Are the Facts of Life," *New York Times*, 7 June 1992, p. A33.

3. "Kaye Brown Houston, 19 Years Old," *Newsweek,* 3 August 1992, p. 46.

4. Steven Seidman, *Embattled Eros: Sexual Politics and Ethics in Contemporary America* (New York: Routledge, 1992), p. 165.

5. Gabrielle Brown, *The New Celibacy: A Journey of Love, Intimacy, and Good Health in a New Age,* 2d ed. (New York: McGraw-Hill, 1989), p. 18.

6. Centers for Disease Control and Prevention, "Sexual Behavior among High School Students—United States, 1990," *Morbidity and Mortality Weekly Report* 40 (January 3, 1992): 885–888. See also Associated Press, "Teen-Agers and AIDS: The Risk Worsens," *New York Times,* 14 April 1992, p. B6.

7. Patricia A. Scollay, Martin Doucett, Margeaux Perry, and Brandy Winterbottom, "AIDS Education of College Students: The Effect of an HIV-Positive Lecturer," *AIDS Education and Prevention* 4, no. 2 (1992): 160–171.

8. Willard Gaylin, *Rediscovering Love* (New York: Penguin, 1986), p. 11.

9. Rebecca Voelker, "From Tobacco to Teen Sex: Applying Anti-smoking Fervor to Reduce High-Risk Behavior among Youth," *American Medical News* 35 (13 April 1992): 4.

10. Immanuel Kant, "Duties toward the Body in Respect of Sexual Impulse," in *Lectures on Ethics,* trans. Louis Infield (Indianapolis: Hackett, 1963), p. 163.

11. Paul R. Fleishman, *The Healing Zone: Religious Issues in Psychotherapy* (New York: Paragon House, 1989), pp. 173, 174.

12. Rollo May, *Love and Will* (New York: Bantam Doubleday Dell, 1969), pp. 41, 42.

13. Cornelis A. M. Rietmeijer, John W. Krebs, Paul M. Feorino, and Franklyn N. Judson, "Condoms as Physical and Chemical Barriers against Immunodeficiency Virus," *Journal of the American Medical Association* 258, no. 12 (1988): 1853.

14. Margaret A. Fischl, Gordon M. Dickinson, Gwendolyn B. Scott, Nancy Klimas, Mary Ann Fletcher, and Wade Parks, "Evaluation of Heterosexual Partners, Children, and Household Contacts of Adults with AIDS," *Journal of the American Medical Association* 257, no. 5 (1987): 640–644.

15. Keith Henry, Michael T. Osterholm, and Kristine L. MacDonald, "Reduction of HIV Transmission by Use of Condoms," Letter to the editor, *American Journal of Public Health* 78, no. 9 (1988): 1244.

16. Board of Trustees, American Medical Association, "Prevention and Control of Acquired Immunodeficiency Syndrome: An Interim Report," *Journal of the American Medical Association* 258 (1987): 2098.

17. Paul J. Feldblum and Judith A. Fortney, "Condoms, Spermicides, and the Transmission of Human Immunodeficiency Virus: A Review of the Literature," *American Journal of Public Health* 78 (1988): 53.

18. Vicki L. Seltzer, Jill Rabin, and Fred Benjamin, "Teenagers' Awareness of the Acquired Immunodeficiency Syndrome and the Impact on Their Sexual Behavior," *Obstetrics and Gynecology* 74 (1989): 58.

19. Richard Gordon, "A Critical Review of the Physics and Statistics of Condoms and Their Role in Individual versus Societal Survival of the AIDS Epidemic," *Journal of Sex and Marital Therapy* 15 (Spring 1989): 23, 24.

20. Ezekiel J. Emanuel and Linda L. Emanuel, "Is Our AIDS Policy Ethical?" *American Journal of Medicine* 83 (1987): 20.

21. Neil D. Broom and Charles E. F. Ricket, "The Ethics of Safe Sex," *New Zealand Medical Journal* 101 (1988): 826.

22. I borrow the metaphor of flight from Max Picard, *The Flight from God*, trans. M. Kuschnitzky (Washington, D.C.: Regnery Gateway, 1951 [original 1934]).

23. C. S. Lewis, *Mere Christianity* (New York: Macmillan, 1952), pp. 78, 81.

24. Søren Kierkegaard, *The Concept of Anxiety: A Simple Psychologically Orienting Deliberation on the Dogmatic Issue of Hereditary Sin*, trans. R. Thomte (Princeton, N.J.: Princeton University Press, 1980 [original 1844]), p. 80.

25. John D'Emilio and Estelle B. Freedman, *Intimate Matters: A History of Sexuality in America* (New York: Harper and Row, 1988), pp. 223, 225.

26. William H. McNeill, *Plagues and Peoples* (New York: Anchor Books, 1976), p. 257.

4

Psychiatry and the Challenge of Religious Toleration

In recent years there has been recognition in the psychiatric community of a need for empirical research on the relation of religion to mental health. Harold G. Koenig systematically reviews a massive empirical literature regarding religion and elderly people, concluding as follows: "In summary, as with life satisfaction, well-being, depression, and anxiety, while the number and quality of studies are limited, older adults' perception of pain, functional status, and satisfaction with health appear to be positively influenced by religious behaviors and attitudes."[1] It is morally imperative that these sources of meaning be respected, and no doubt they are by the psychiatric profession generally. To ensure this respect, in 1990 the American Psychiatric Association approved a set of ethical guidelines that warns against the imposition of "antireligious or ideologic systems of beliefs" on patients, and requires that "psychiatrists should maintain respect for their patients' beliefs."[2]

But there are some expressions of religion, particularly in its intense or novel forms, that truly challenge the tolerance of even the most tolerant psychiatrist. This chapter is no apology for destructive forms of religious belief or practice; however, if we are to take the American constitutional tradition of religious free exercise seriously, forms of religion that are socially unpopular and controversial must not become the target of psychiatric inquisition. The principal focus of this chapter is the psychiatric response to the various new religious movements (NRMs) that emerged in American society in the late 1960s and early 1970s. But before turning to this topic, I will comment on some broader related concerns.

POSSIBLE NEGATIVE BIAS

Bias against women, homosexuals, and racial minorities has been of concern to psychiatry, as demonstrated by a willingness to revise or delete diagnostic categories and definitions of mental illness when appropriate.[3] Objectivity, that is, the absence of all bias, is of course an ideal that is never fully reached, because psychiatry like any other discipline has its own particular worldview, which is both historical and interpretive. Still, because psychiatry is so powerful socially and politically, it should avoid the pretense of objectivity in controversial areas of nosology (definition of mental illness) and acknowledge that its interpretation of some phenomena may be reductionistic or erroneous.

Reductive interpretations of religious phenomena inevitably lead to insensitivity and lack of empathy toward those persons who manifest particular beliefs and behaviors of a religious nature. My concern here is with unintended negative bias that stems from insensitivity and that can harm the therapeutic effort of the psychiatrist when dealing with religious people. Of course empathy has limits. A secular psychiatrist justifiably refuses to pray with a patient who requests prayer, for example.

I believe that there may be some evidence of negative bias in the official nomenclature of American psychiatry, *Diagnostic and Statistical Manual of Mental Disorders,* third edition revised, called DSM-III-R.[4] DSM-III-R is an influential document used as a standard for diagnoses and training in American psychiatry. It is the product of generations of effort to clarify and write the definitions of psychopathology, and it has important societal consequences both here and abroad, having been translated into more than a dozen foreign languages. DSM-III-R attempts to avoid empirically unjustified diagnostic constructs, although concepts of illness are inevitably relative to a socially dominant image of normal behavior. It is diagnostically conservative in the sense that it generally defines in detail the criteria that a patient must fulfill before being placed in a disease category. The manual is reasonably sensitive to the importance of diagnoses with regard to treatment, law, institutionalization, social stigma, the self-concept of the individual who is diagnosed, and basic human rights. Nevertheless, it leaves something to be desired with respect to religion.

The "Glossary of Technical Terms" included in DSM-III-R is a case in point. The possibility of "negative religious bias" in DSM-III (the unrevised version of the third edition) and DSM-III-R was first highlighted in 1984 by James T. Richardson, a sociologist.[5] An unnecessary accumulation of religious examples of pathology in the glossary gives the impression that religion is indicative of illness. The examples are presented under "catatonic posturing," "delusion," "delusion of being controlled," "delusion (grandiose)," "hallucination (tactile)," "illogical thinking," "incoherence," "magical thinking," "mood-congruent psychotic features," "mood-incongruent psychotic features," and "poverty of content of speech."

With regard to religious experience, the glossary lists "special relationship to a deity" as an instance of "mood-congruent psychotic features." A suspicion is cast upon persons who feel a proximity to God or the gods. It can certainly be said that persons who suffer from either a depressed or manic mood might feel a "special relationship to a deity." Moreover, this entry does not make religion the only framework in which such psychotic features occur. A patient might feel a special relationship to "a famous person" such as a political leader, rather than to the deity. But more critically, does psychiatry understand that believers in most religious traditions teach nothing short of a "special" and intimate relationship with the deity? If a patient expressed an intense feeling of "special" proximity to God, would this be suspect?

Perhaps a more convincing case for bias in DSM-III-R can be made from the "Magical Thinking" entry. In order to provide the reader with a context, the paragraphs are fully quoted:

> The person believes that his or her thoughts, words, or actions might, or will in some manner, cause or prevent a specific outcome in some way that defies the normal laws of cause and effect. Example: A man believed that if he said a specific prayer three times each night, his mother's death might be prevented indefinitely: a mother believed that if she had an angry thought, her child would become ill.
>
> Magical thinking may be part of ideas of reference or may reach delusional proportions when the person maintains a firm conviction about the belief despite evidence to the contrary.

Magical thinking is seen in children, in primitive cultures, and in Schizotypal Personality Disorder, Schizophrenia, and Obsessive Compulsive Disorder.

The above passages are complex because prayer is placed in the context of "delusional proportions" and "evidence to the contrary." The writers also place prayer in the context of "magical thinking." It is easy to assume that "magical thinking" is somewhat distinct from mere imagination, that it implies a proneness toward fantasy—if not psychopathology—in violation of what might be generally termed the "reality principle" as the empirical tradition of secular psychiatry defines it.

These passages are further complicated because the man prays for the "indefinite" prevention of his mother's death. "Indefinite" need not imply "infinite." We all know that the infinite prevention of death is impossible. But an "indefinite" period generally refers to a period of undefined length that will eventually come to an end, and therefore does not violate empirical possibility.

Finally, prayer is set in the context of the number three, which may be intended to indicate some odd superstitious fetish. It is common knowledge, however, that in many traditions, prayers are said in repetition. The Roman Catholic rosary, for example, is a string of beads containing sets of five, fifteen, and three, used to keep count of prayers. Buddhism also uses beads to keep count of chants. The patient in question here is possibly steeped in Catholic piety, in contrast to Protestant. Are Catholics more likely to be labeled mentally ill because of the more ritualistic aspects of their tradition?

Would a prayer in a different context not indicate psychopathology? Would a prayer for the health of an ill mother with reference neither to the number three nor to "indefinite" preservation of life be an example of an acceptable religious practice? DSM-III-R omits any reference to the possibility of sane prayer. Is prayer suspect?

According to DSM-III-R, the continuation of prayer despite "evidence to the contrary" is indicative of psychopathology. But religious traditions define faith as the very willingness to maintain "firm conviction" even when there is reason to give up hope. Faith transcends "evidence to the contrary," or it is not faith.

Especially derogatory is the association made under "magical think-ing" between a person who prays and "children" or "people in primitive cultures." Religious persons are thereby infantilized and ridiculed as prim-itive. (People in primitive cultures are, by implication, childish and crazy.) This ridicule applies to the more than 90 percent of the American people reported to believe in God and the efficacy of prayer by the Gallop study on the theme "Religion in America."[6] Presumably they would prefer to think that effective prayer has a place in the life of a modern and sophisti-cated adult. That prayer is viewed with such suspicion in DSM-III-R may be loosely associated with the fact that, as of the last formal survey, only 40 percent of psychiatrists profess a belief in God.[7]

Another entry in the glossary that may demonstrate insensitivity–and tastelessness–is "Catatonic Posturing," because the only example provided is a patient who "may stand with arms outstretched as if he were Jesus on the cross." DSM-III-R could provide alternative examples, unless the reader is to assume that this illness occurs exclusively among religious per-sons. One wonders if it is understood that many religious traditions include particular forms of body posturing in their ritual and worship.

DSM-III-R is also questionable in its treatment of religious thought. In the glossary, under "Poverty of Content of Speech," the following is entered:

Speech that is adequate in amount but conveys little information because of vagueness, empty repetitions, or use of stereotyped or obscure phrases. The interviewer may observe that the person has spoken at some length, but has not given adequate information to answer a question. Alternatively, the person may provide enough information to answer the question, but require many words to do so, so that his or her lengthy reply can be summarized in a sentence or two. The expression *poverty of content of speech* is generally not used when speech is, for the most part, not understandable (incoherence). Example: Interviewer: "O.K. Why is it, do you think, that people believe in God?" Patient: "Well, first of all because, He is the person that, is their personal savior. He walks with me and talks with me. And uh, the understanding that I have, a lot of peoples, they don't really know their own personal self. Because they ain't, they all, just don't know their own personal self. They don't know that He uh, seemed like to me, a lot of em don't understand that He walks and talks with them. And uh, show 'em their way to go. I understand also that, every man and every lady, is just not pointed in the same direction. Some are pointed different. They go in their different ways. The way that Jesus Christ wanted 'em to go. Myself, I am pointed in the ways of uh, knowing right from wrong, and doing it. I can't do any more, or not less than that."

This example is the only one offered, and it is unnecessarily (but predictably) specific to religion. It could imply for those who do not know better that a religious worldview is typically accepted by persons psychopathically incapable of logical and persuasive speech. (Incidentally, the reference to "lengthy reply" that could be summarized "in a sentence or two" describes many academics.)

Yet the above passage does not indicate poverty of content of speech; they are rather developed statements in the dialect of a particular social group. The principal bias could thus be other than religious. Such passages can easily be translated into meaningful phrases acceptable to the culture of the interviewer. The patient responds roughly as follows:

People believe in God, first of all, because they feel that God is their personal savior. They feel this deeply and intimately. Of course, some people don't really understand themselves very well. They don't understand how close they can be to God personally, and that God can show them the way to go in their lives. And of course I realize that people are different, and they aren't all pointed in the same direction. They go their different ways. But as for myself, I go the way of Christ, with a clear desire to do the right rather than the wrong morally. I can do nothing more, nothing less.

Arguably, the unwillingness of the interviewer to see the reasonableness in these passages indicates cultural and class insensitivities. But bias against religious images of human fulfillment could also result in the unwillingness to undertake the obvious task of translation.

Second, one wonders why the interviewer would pose such an intellectually challenging question to test for content of speech. Trained philosophers and theologians have struggled to say why they believe in God. The very difficulty of the question makes it inappropriate as a test for "content of speech," particularly when presented to the ordinary religious believer for whom God is more likely "felt" than abstractly defined. The interviewer should have posed a simple mundane question or else assessed speech content in the process of general conversation with the patient.

The question is repeated in the glossary under "Incoherence." The interviewer asks, "Why do you think people believe in God?" Again, the patient does his or her best with a complex question that would catch anyone off guard. The interviewer might have proceeded thus: "Why do you think people believe in psychotherapy?"

In its defense, I must add that DSM-III-R does state that it intends to avoid bias. In the glossary, immediately after the entry "Magical Thinking," is this passage under "Mental Disorder": "Neither deviant behavior, e.g., political, religious, or sexual, nor conflicts that are primarily between the individual and society are mental disorders unless the deviance or conflict is a symptom of a dysfunction in the person as described above." The introduction to DSM-III-R also includes a cautionary statement. Still, if prayer itself is suspect as childish and primitive, and if theism is incoherent, then this warning is not very reassuring.

DSM-III-R AND NEW RELIGIOUS MOVEMENTS

According to its own warning, DSM-III-R does not want to label and stigmatize nonconformist religious behavior that is primarily a conflict between individual and society. Consistent with this laudable commitment, the American Psychiatric Association has taken up some of the many ethical issues that psychiatry faces regarding religion. This is especially evident in its evenhanded review of the problem of social bias against members of new religious movements—or of religious groups that are old in Asia and other parts of world but newly imported into the United States.

Through its Committee on Psychiatry and Religion (at the request of its board of trustees), chaired by Marc Galanter, a psychiatrist, *Cults and New Religious Movements: A Report of the American Psychiatric Association* was published in 1989. This report is the culmination of a three-year project designed to assess NRMs and the proper role, if any, of psychiatry in addressing them. Galanter writes in the preface that the report allows divergent and often conflicting views to be presented and leaves the reader to develop his or her own perspectives.[8]

Several authors contributing to the report put DSM-III-R under considerable critical scrutiny for its passages on "cultists." A vague and dangerous passage in DSM-III-R, according to these several authors, is found in the chapter entitled "Dissociative Disorders," under section 300.15, "Dissociative Disorder Not Otherwise Specified." The fifth disorder listed in 300.15 is this: "(5) dissociated states that may occur in people who have been subjected to periods of prolonged and intense coercive persuasion (e.g., brainwashing, thought reform, or indoctrination while the captive of terrorists or cultists)." "May occur" means that dissociation does not always occur. But nevertheless DSM-III-R places its weighty imprimatur on a set of stereotypes that are already, in the popular culture, "highly resistant to inconsistent and contradictory evidence."[9] One wonders if accusation of "brainwashing" is the modern equivalent of the medieval charge that heretics are "bewitched."

The Ethics Committee of the American Psychiatric Association, in its "Opinions," writes that joining a "new religion" is not in itself evidence of mental illness.[10] This statement is a fair one because it does not use the derogatory term "cult," nor does it presuppose that members of NRMs are mentally ill. It does, however, seem to be at odds with DSM-III-R 300.15 (5), which lumps "cultists" and "terrorists" together in the same category and presumes that a person does not freely join an NRM because of an attraction to its worldview but, rather, is held physically captive and then "brainwashed." Yet opponents of NRMs have only very rarely alleged that recruits are physically captive, an essential condition for "brainwashing" to occur as it is defined by Robert Jay Lifton and others.[11] If incarceration were present, the legal system would long ago have put an end to the practice, for no one believes that the freedom to recruit religious converts extends to kidnapping and forced confinement.

Section 300:15 (5) of DSM-III-R is included in the chapter on "Dissociative Disorders." As DSM-III-R defines such disorders, they involve patients for whom "customary identity is temporarily forgotten," a "new identity may be assumed or imposed," and the "customary feeling of one's own reality is lost and replaced by a feeling of unreality." Thus DSM-III-R creates an image of the member of an NRM as not his or her authentic self but rather as dissociated from the main mental system that constitutes the normal conscious personality. This implies that people who join NRMs are not active and psychologically integrated agents purposely experimenting with a set of new religious teachings but instead are "zombies" passively "bewitched" and no longer "themselves." This is a stereotype, and judging from its "Opinions," the American Psychiatric Association does not really want to endorse it. Throughout history, any individual who has undergone intense religious conversion, that is, the intellectual and emotional migration from one worldview to another, has appeared very different from his or her former self because in fact the self has changed in a way that puts it at odds with its previous social environment.

It is evident that members of NRMs are frequently stimuli of dread and panic to some people, especially worried parents. In the Galanter report, the psychiatrist Saul V. Levine worries about the use of the term "cultist" for just this reason. He notes the following: "We must bear in mind, however, that the label cult is partly in the eye of the beholder, and that a remarkable array of groups has had that eponym applied to them. Groups that this author has heard called cults by concerned relatives of members have included Catholics, Mormons, Orthodox Jewry, Born Again Christians, Bahai, IBM, est, and Gestalt, to name but a few."[12] DSM-III-R introduces the word "cultist" into official nomenclature for the first time, without offering any definition whatsoever, and without caution.

Is a new religious movement a "cult" because of the presence of a powerful charismatic leader who has authority over a convert's life? If so, then nearly all significant religions, at points in their history, would qualify. From Jesus to the Prophet Mohammed, from John Wesley to Mother Ann Lee of the Shakers, religious founders and leaders have made demands specific to every aspect of human experience and desire.

Is it the degree of self-surrender that defines a cult? Daily self-denial, devotion, and discipline are characteristic of all religious life in its more serious forms. The very word "Islam" derives from the Arabic root for surrender, resignation, and peace. As Larry R. Shinn, a historian of Asian religions, writes, "Most religious traditions of the world ideally require complete dedication to the life and worldview that their founders and sages have espoused."[13] Even a cursory glance at Hindu teachings on the relationship between guru and disciple, or Christian teachings on the relationship between novitiate and monastic superior, reveals that intense religious persons are willing to deny voluntarily what to them is a false individuality corrupted by the lack of religious meaning.

Presumably most psychiatrists do not take kindly to the undifferentiated name-calling that contributes to the ghettoization of religious communities and perhaps to their consequent persecution. On the basis of DSM-III-R, however, some mental health "experts" have labeled religious converts "brainwashed" in legal proceedings without ever having interviewed them. As has been pointed out in the Galanter report, "Of interest to the mental health profession is the curious fact that, in a surprisingly large number of deprogramming cases, professionals, including psychiatrists, have supported applications for conservatorships based upon purported conclusions of the mental ill health of a proposed conservatee who had never been examined."[14]

In a number of "brainwashing" cases, DSM-III and DSM-III-R have been offered to the courts to substantiate such testimony. A full discussion of these court cases is beyond the scope of this chapter, but I mention them to indicate the severe conflict between the religious nonconformist and society.

Some psychiatrists, for example John G. Clark, see in religious conversions to NRMs only involuntary, trancelike states of dissociation and complete loss of control over one's mind.[15] But nonetheless, every mystic, Eastern or Western, from Buddha to the poet William Blake, has spoken of a path to liberation from the chains of ordinary consciousness through the free denial of the false self in order ultimately to discover the true self in its genuineness. As Harvey Cox, one of America's foremost theologians, has written:

> Some psychiatrists contend that young people who join Oriental religious movements or Jesus communes have obviously been "brainwashed" since they now share their money and have lost interest in becoming business executives. That someone could freely choose a

path of mystical devotion, self-sacrifice, and the sharing of worldly goods seems self-evidently impossible to them. They forget that . . . according to the Gospel of Mark, Jesus was a candidate for "deprogramming," since his own family thought he was berserk and his religious leaders said he was possessed by the devil.[16]

Of course in a society such as our own, with its laissez faire and anomic individualism, and its radical suspicion of trust in authority, those who reject "normal" career goals and relations in order freely to devote themselves to an intense religious vocation are going to be labeled "slave," "robot," "programmed," and now, by DSM-III-R, "dissociated." This constitutes the medicalization of nonconformity in the religious sphere.

Religious commitment will be explained away with platitudes—"She was lonely and without direction," or "His family life was never quite adequate." Thus what is often a potent form of self-determination is conveniently reduced to vulnerability and passive manipulation. The psychiatrist Louis Jolyon West, in his contribution to the Galanter report, attacks "cults" primarily because members supposedly lose personal freedom.[17] But contrary to West's thought, believers themselves respond that their lifestyle is taken up wholeheartedly and that their choice of a disciplined and devotional life is an expression of religious desires.

The authority of charismatic leaders can be a force for good or for bad. Charismatic movements are a perennial feature of human experience, and many have contributed to, or even resulted in the creation of, the great centers of world culture. Some have indeed been destructive. But this uncertainty is an inevitable aspect of many spheres of human experience from universities to family life, from politics to business, from medicine to law. The First Amendment provides for the free exercise of religion without claiming that religion is any more free of risk than these other areas.

There are charismatic groups that have violated the autonomy of the religious seeker and inflicted harms. There was the Peoples' Temple, a Christian-socialist evangelical community (not a NRM) that turned to incarceration and regulated terror and eventually to murder and mass suicide in the deplorable Jonestown Massacre. Here the legal system must prosecute to the fullest, just as it does in any other social context when the laws have been violated. It is the existing law, and not vicious innuendo, that should set limits to religious behavior. Parents unwilling to relinquish control over their adult children's lives are not the ones to set these limits; often great religious leaders have suffered intense resistance from family members. I do think that parents ought to have greater control over their children's religious commitments when the children are legally minors.

Unfortunately, there is no way of knowing ahead of time which charismatic movements—political, religious, or social—will prove destructive of freedom and well-being. Some movements die out, some make a significant positive contribution to society in time. We only know them by their fruits.

Anti-"cult" literature has made effective use of the 1978 events at Jonestown, Guyana, by lumping virtually all NRMs together into what Shinn dubs the "Jonestown Syndrome." As Shinn comments, "These tendencies to exaggerate the similarities and dangers of all the cults have been two major forces in promoting public suspicion and fear of such groups."[18] In the Galanter report, West advocates a "public health" approach to all NRMs, because "most—if not all—have the potential of becoming deadly, as the People's Temple of Jim Jones did."[19] In point of fact, we have not seen this epidemic of death and destruction. Nearly all the NRMs of the 1960s and 1970s have quietly declined as a result of high attrition (a fact that "deprogrammers" and angry parents selectively ignore), and not one has become a second Jonestown, with the possible exception of a small band of Branch Davidians in Waco, Texas.

In a systematic and controlled study of one new religion, the Unification Church, Eileen Barker, a professor of sociology at the London School of Economics, concludes that of the few potential recruits who, after an introductory evening lecture, decide to attend a weekend retreat either in England or the United States, less than 12 percent stay on and join this church. Within a year, one-third of these recruits leave the movement, and afterward attrition rates are as high as 75 percent.[20] Recruits are free to leave, and they do, Barker concludes. Many only joined to experiment with a new religion that they eventually reject. Of the Hare Krishnas, Shinn writes that "of the more than nine thousand devotees that Prabhupada [founder of the International Society for Krishna Consciousness (ISKCON), or Hare Krishna] initiated, fewer than two thousand remain in ISKCON."[21] These careful studies explode the myth that members of these two movements are held captive, unable to "escape" without the "aid" of "deprogrammers." There are no significant continuities between enthusiastic religious proselytizers with their songs, prayers, and public lectures, and violent terrorists. Terrorism should not be confused with religious enthusiasm, a strong esprit de corps, and close-knit community, from which even the truest believers often walk away.

In the Galanter report, Galanter cites research indicating that only those who have been "deprogrammed," that is, coercively removed from their NRMs and resocialized in an attempt to get them to "renounce their beliefs and accept more traditional ones," are the ones who promulgate the captivity stories. As Galanter concludes, "Those who left voluntarily retained a notable fidelity to the sect, in contrast to those who were deprogrammed."[22] Those who leave NRMs on their own do not create the atrocity tales, although they may be disappointed that their experiment with salvation came to naught. Researchers who study NRMs should not base their conclusions only on the accounts of disaffected "deprogrammed" former members alone but also on the accounts of active NRM members and on those of the large numbers of former members who freely passed through the revolving door. Would we base our assessment of marriage solely on the account of coercively divorced people subjected under "deprogramming" to physical incarceration and antimarriage ideology?

The phrase "while the captive of terrorists or cultists" is not the only one in DSM-III-R 300.15 (5) filled with misleading innuendos. The terms "coercive persuasion," "brainwashing," and "thought reform," are equally problematic. The psychiatrists J. Thomas Ungerleider and David K. Wellisch write in the Galanter report as follows: "But unlike most conditions listed in DSM-III *no* signs, symptoms, or other criteria for diagnosis are listed! No psychological tests exist that diagnose the syndrome of coercive persuasion and we have found no indication of overt mental illness in our cult population study."[23] Brock K. Kilbourne, another contributor to the Galanter report, describes DSM-III-R 300.15 (5) as "vague and incomplete in diagnostic information, lacking in established reliability and validity, confused conceptually with brainwashing and terrorism, and does not specify how new religious affiliation results in dissociated

states."[24] If these authors are correct, then DSM-III-R 300.15 (5) reflex-
ively assigns patients associated with unpopular religious movements to a
diagnostic gray box.[25]

Although I strongly disagree with Thomas Szasz's antipsychiatry thesis that all mental illness, including severe forms, is a myth, Szasz, a psychiatrist himself, does take a useful stance on "brainwashing": "A person
can no more wash another's brain with coercion or conversation than he
can make him bleed with a cutting remark. If there is no such thing as
brainwashing, what does the metaphor stand for? It stands for one of the
most universal human experiences and events, namely, for one person
influencing another. However, we do not call all types of personal or psychological influence 'brainwashing.' We reserve this term for influence of
which we disapprove."[26]

Whether "brainwashing" is merely a term of opprobrium is a question worth considering. Outside of a physically coercive environment,
such as that described in Lifton's study of American soldiers subjected to
hsi-nao ("wash brain") by the Chinese in the Korean War period, one
doubts if the term has any significance. Under physical coercion and the
threat of bodily harm, perhaps some persons can be forced to change their
worldviews, although if this occurs, one wonders why they so quickly
reject the ideology of their captors upon liberation.

But assuming brainwashing can occur under the conditions of physical coercion or the threat of such, it is inconsistent to remove these conditions in an effort to extend the brainwashing metaphor into the domain
of time-honored religious conversions. The teaching of notions of a divine
judge, of heaven and hell, and of the need to experience salvation are
essential to almost all religious traditions and are routinely rejected or
accepted freely by persons with varying needs. If the extension of brainwashing is allowed, then any significant reform of a person's thoughts and
habits through education, persuasive argument, and socialization is suspect. Phenomenologically, persons are constantly subjected to efforts at
reform both of thought and behavior. The intensity of a medical school
curriculum is designed to make willing participants think and feel differently about a wide variety of phenomena. Were students forced to
undergo this process of reform unwillingly, and without possibility of
escape, then medical schools would have to be condemned. Persons con-

stantly induce others to behave or think differently by persuasive means, ranging from public lectures to intense private argument. New religious movements provide arguments through presentation of theological world-views. Proselytizers surely are aware that potential recruits have basic human needs for affirmation, a sense of community, and of purpose. But this does not make religious movements any different from social clubs and college fraternities.

Moreover, as the sociologist James T. Richardson points out in the Galanter report, the recruit who considers joining a new religion is "work-ing out" a search for meaning, and thus "actively contributing to his or her induction." Human beings are "meaning-seeking entities" who pursue "creative transformations."[27] This model of agency in the context of reli-gious conversion is, according to Richardson, now dominant among humanistic social scientists. More behaviorally oriented social scientists will not take the view that, as Carl Jung suggested, the modern self is "in search of a soul." It is largely the behaviorists, who hold that we are all "beyond freedom and dignity," who have applied the unfortunate meta-phor of "programming" to religious persons. Lowell D. Streiker, former executive director of Freedom Counseling Center, an agency assisting individuals and families disturbed by "cults," writes of the "few expert wit-nesses of the anticult movement" as follows:

> The alleged "sophisticated techniques of thought reform" about which they warn us are, in fact, the ordinary means of persuasion and social influence which are freely used by established religions, civic organizations, political parties, salespeople, the media and advertisers. If it were as easy to deprive individuals of their free will and retain them as zealous participants as the anticult movements' experts sug-gest, every man, woman, or child would long since have succumbed to the siren of the so-called cults.[28]

Streiker points out how the numbers of NRMs, as well as their sizes, have been badly exaggerated by the anti-"cultists."

The matter of NRMs is just one branch on a large tree. If our society is to avoid religious intolerance and future inquisitions, we will have to be more careful than ever about how controversial religious practices are labeled. The recent report from the Committee on Psychiatry and Religion, from which this chapter has drawn for criticism of DSM-III-R section 300.15(5), is an advance.

It would be helpful if psychiatrists such as Saul V. Levine could be heard above the rhetoric. Levine describes the experiences of many members of NRMs as follows: "The vast majority of members go through these experiences relatively unscathed, have a tough time after they (almost inevitably) come out (usually in under two years), and gradually reconstitute and reintegrate. For most of the youthful members, the radical departure ends up as an intense life experience that few people would have recommended or prescribed, but which manages to serve a developmental purpose." So long as laws are not broken, "all manner of intense group belief systems have to be tolerated" in a "democratic society," concludes Levine.[29]

Another psychiatrist, Paul C. Mohl, asks psychiatrists to ponder this: "Any sweeping generalizations about cults, cult members, and cult practices run the risk of reflecting the psychiatrist's personal bias, not his or her truly expert professional opinion." Mohl adds an historical note: "I found myself wondering how I would have regarded the Mormons in the 1830s." Most important, Mohl provides this practical suggestion for clinical psychiatrists: "It is probably a good idea for the psychiatrist to ask, 'Would I support hospital commitment of this patient if I were unaware of the cult membership.'"[30] Some psychiatrists may need this advice.

The sad results of a growing intolerance against innocent religious groups are now with us. Franklin H. Littell, one of the foremost scholars in the area of religious liberties, describes one incident: "In July 1988 the newspapers carried the story of Mary Susan Greve, formerly Sister Mary Cecelia of the St. Joseph Novitiate Convent, a dissident Roman Catholic group in Roundtop, New York. Miss Greve was kidnapped out of her training center, with her family claiming the convent was a 'cult.' Apparently the family pressure won out, for she now claims she was 'brainwashed' by the convent and its spiritual leader."[31] Does DSM-III-R provide the diagnostic category that might justify such actions? that might convince courts to rule uncritically on behalf of disaffected former members of virtually any religious community? that might place a damper on the hitherto protected right of religious communities to proselytize? Littell's warning is especially pointed: "The danger to religious liberty in

America today—in contrast to earlier generations—comes not so much from vigilantes as from self-styled 'scientists' who have surrounded their hostility to religion with a whole set of 'scientific' claims about religion, about personality, about the life of the mind, about ultimate values and truth."[32] If Littell's assessment is accurate, it may be that an effort to remedy the inconsistencies in DSM-III-R will only begin to solve the underlying hostility to religion and NRMs.

PSYCHIATRY AND "DEPROGRAMMING"

David Bromley and Anson Shupe, two prominent sociologists studying deprogramming, describe deprogrammings inflicted on adult converts to new religious movements, on Mormons, on Old Catholics, on charismatic Episcopalians, and on Christian evangelicals, among others, all made possible through psychiatric testimonies leading to parental removal of the rights of adult children to freedom of movement through conservatorships.[33] Some deprogramming cases involved converts to radical political beliefs. For example, Susan Wirth, who held a doctoral degree in Spanish literature, was handcuffed to a bed for two weeks and denied food. Why? "Wirth's mother did not approve of her radical political beliefs and paid [Ted] Patrick $27,000 to make her 'normal.'"[34] A case that captured national attention was the abduction of Stephanie Reithmiller in 1981. Deprogrammers were hired by her parents, who "objected to their adult daughter's living with another woman in an alleged lesbian relationship."[35] There was no known psychiatric involvement in these latter two cases.

How extensive has psychiatric involvement in the deprogramming movement been? Lee Coleman, a psychiatrist who opposes his colleagues' making religious converts forcibly available to deprogrammers through supporting conservatorships, produced the definitive historical statement. It begins thus: "When I argue that psychiatry has become a weapon in a holy war against certain religions, I will not thereby be supporting the goals or doctrines of any of these organizations. Neither will I be attacking them. Rather, I am suggesting that psychiatry has absolutely no business influencing a person's religious preference or determining whether a religion is valid or bogus." Coleman, with a wealth of documentation, contends that for the deprogramming movement, "psychiatry became crucial to the cause."[36] It was the major source of legal legitimation through conservatorship proceedings, especially after kidnapping of religious converts off street corners or out of ashrams began to draw criticism.

Coleman provides the now folkloric case of Wes Lockwood, a student at Yale University who joined Hannah Lowe's New Testament Missionary Fellowship. His Catholic father was irate and hired the infamous Ted Patrick to kidnap and deprogram his son. The young Lockwood struggled against his captors as the group drove down the highway, drawing the attention of the state highway patrol. Coleman cites from Patrick's own book, "Fortunately, Lockwood Sr. was carrying a letter from the Yale Psychiatric Department and this had a most dramatic softening effect on the attitude of the troopers."[37] Coleman gives numerous other examples.

In 1980, with the support of anticult psychiatrists, Howard Lasker, a member of the New York State Assembly, introduced an amendment to the state's mental hygiene law, stating that people known to have undergone religious conversion and subsequent personality change would be automatically subject to forty-five days of "psychological and/or psychiatric treatment."[38] Governor Hugh Carey refused to sign the bill. No other states have successfully introduced such a bill.

Coleman complains that the profession of psychiatry has looked the other way regarding psychiatric abuse in the area of religious conversion. Agencies outside of psychiatry have not. "For example," he writes, "the Massachusetts Board of Registration and Discipline in Medicine (Medical Licensing Board) investigated Dr. Clark for his role in the Ed Shapiro [deprogramming] affair." The board concluded that Clark's diagnosis of Shapiro was "based entirely on the subject's religion," offered a clear-cut rebuke of Clark, but took no formal action.[39]

Elizabeth Rogow, a Columbia University student, and hundreds of other adult converts to sects of various sorts, from fundamentalist Christians to Jews for Jesus, "fell victim to the hospitalization tactic." Pam Fanshier, a college graduate, was involuntarily committed to the psychiatric ward at Central Kansas Medical Center, but "was given official clearance by the psychiatrists, who formally proclaimed her to be without mental disorder and not dangerous to herself or others. Had she been a feisty type, . . . the outcome might have been quite different."[40]

In presenting this brief history, I have avoided as much as possible any naming of psychiatrists. A chapter such as this one, however, would be rightly rejected were the historical events left undocumented. Psychiatric abuse in the context of deprogramming far outstrips that found to have taken place in the witch-hunts of the 1930s against political leftists, such as the actress Francis Farmer. That even a few psychiatrists could become directly active in an inquisition against socially unaccepted religious beliefs is of concern.

Yet the authors of an authoritative study of religion and psychology consider "brainwashing" models to be "tools of personal rhetoric legitimating political suppression of unpopular religious groups." They conclude that despite the controversy surrounding NRMs, the study of religious conversions "requires a less polemical analysis of what is a more general process rooted firmly in the history of religion."[41] To reiterate, reductive behavioristic analyses of religious conversion displaced the emphasis on personal narratives of conversion experience characteristic of classical studies such as William James's *Varieties of Religious Experience,* published in 1902.

CONCLUDING CONCERNS

We must be sufficiently tolerant to distinguish genuine harm from unfounded vicious innuendo. Scholars in the area of church and state have long counseled caution against religious bigotry. Anson Stokes and Leo Pfeffer, writing three decades ago, recalled the convent controversies of 1834. A young woman named Harrison "began telling lurid tales of her convent life. These stirred up much public indignation, strengthened by reports in the Boston newspapers." Extreme anti-Catholic sermons followed. Harrison returned to the Ursuline Convent outside of Boston. The city selectmen visited the convent to see for themselves that she was not enchained. They issued a report that Harrison was there of her free will, but it was too late to prevent catastrophe. A mob burned the convent as they shouted "No Popery." They believed her "to have been placed in some dungeon."[42] It is important to learn from the Boston selectmen— form opinions based on fact rather than prejudice.

Every society has its tyranny of the normal, defended by "experts." Our highly individualistic and essentially secular image of the self truly is, as Lifton points out, a product of the Renaissance. The free mind is defined as one at liberty to explore without the fear of losing faith or of punishment. Unaided human reason must replace all submission to religious authority. Humanism brought back to the minds of Europeans the daring critical and questioning habits of the ancient philosophers, habits that some argue have been the inspiration of creative genius and progress in freedom ever since. One fruit of this new freedom was the expression of the individual self and individual whim. Against this backdrop, members of many sects and religious communities appear excessively under control, especially to outsiders. But is this backdrop inevitably distorting? Must we all reject serious religious authority in order to be judged sane?

Underlying the tendency to widen the definition of "brainwashing" in order to encompass commitment to doctrinaire and enthusiastic political and religious groups is a value bias against deeply serious believers. The psychiatrist E. Fuller Torrey points out that psychiatry is culture and class bound, associated with middle-class values such as self-reliance, individualism, enhancement of wealth and social status, and rationalism.[43] The many forms of religious devotion, self-denial, and spiritual discipline that reject these values are bound to prove offensive.

Lifton clearly reveals the value base of psychiatry when he writes that his concern is with "totalism, or what I would call fundamentalism." What he "would describe as a worldwide epidemic of fundamentalism in its political, religious, or combined forms" is, he writes, especially disturbing. Why so disturbing? Because fundamentalism rejects "a liberating dimension of Western history that has evolved, with great struggle, pain, and conflict, from the time of the Renaissance."[44] To reject such individualism, which is so excessive when measured against most cultures and histories, is by his definition to be unhealthy. Yet clearly fundamentalism is the endeavor to reconstruct secular society according to the dictates of traditional religions in which the individual is subservant to the community.

Modernity, at a decent moral minimum, should not *impose* the liberal norm of individualism and anomie on those who find its liberating powers shallow and unconvincing. Lifton is aware of this, as his remarks on so-called deprogramming imply: "Totalism begets totalism—and there can be notable totalism in so-called deprogramming. . . . My own position, which I have stated many times and have conveyed to parents and others who have consulted me, is that I am against coercion at either end of the cult process."[45] Lifton, while devoted to the development of individualism in the Renaissance and Enlightenment traditions, fortunately does not want to force religious converts to be "free" as he narrowly defines freedom. Instead, he advocates educational efforts against "totalist" currents. Here I agree with him.

Any thorough discussion of a psychiatric role in the legal restraint of religious conversion in general must contain a historical note. The youthful medieval converts to the Dominicans and Franciscans were called *dementes* ("insane") by the establishment. Both Saint Francis and Saint Thomas Aquinas were kidnapped and imprisoned for lengthy periods of time by their parents and relatives, who tried to "deprogram" them away from their novel beliefs. Saint Thomas wrote a remarkable treatise—*Contra pestiferam doctrinam retrahentium homines a religionis ingressu*, or, "Against the Pernicious Teaching of Those Dragging Youth Away from Entering the Religious Life."

Free exercise of religion as guaranteed by the First Amendment is permissive regarding what appear to be eccentric religious beliefs and practices, but all believers who violate laws are to be subjected to the full weight of the judicial system. Free exercise of religion is a bit risky, but all necessary freedoms carry the possibility for misuse. The only alternative to religious free exercise is the draconian control of individual religious conscience and the state imprimatur on persecution.

NOTES

1. Harold G. Koenig, "Research on Religion and Mental Health in Later Life: A Review and Commentary," *Journal of Geriatric Psychiatry* 123, no. 1 (1990): 39.

2. American Psychiatric Association, "Guidelines Regarding Possible Conflict between Psychiatrists' Religious Commitments and Psychiatric Practice," *American Journal of Psychiatry* 147 (1990): 542.

3. Ronald Bayer, *Homosexuality and American Psychiatry: The Politics of Diagnosis* (Princeton, N.J.: Princeton University Press, 1979).

4. *Diagnostic and Statistical Manual of Mental Disorders: (third edition revised): DSM-III-R* (Washington, D.C.: American Psychiatric Association, 1987).

5. James T. Richardson, "Negative Religious Bias in the DSM-III and the DSM-III-R" (Paper presented at a meeting of the Society for the Social-Scientific Study of Religion, Chicago, 1984).

6. George Gallop, Jr., *Gallop Opinion Index: Religion in America* (Princeton, N.J.: American Institute of Public Opinion, Princeton University, 1981).

7. *American Psychiatric Association Task Force Report 10: Psychiatrist's Viewpoints on Religion and Their Services to Religious Institutions and the Ministry* (Washington, D.C.: American Psychiatric Association, 1975).

8. Marc M. Galanter, Preface, in Marc M. Galanter, ed., *Cults and New Religious Movements: A Report of the American Psychiatric Association from the Committee on Psychiatry and Religion* (Washington, D.C.: American Psychiatric Association, 1989), pp. xiv, 8.

9. Brock K. Kilbourne and James T. Richardson, "Cultphobia," *Thought Quarterly Review* 61 (1986): 258–266.

10. Opinions of the Ethics Committee on the Principles of Medical Ethics (Washington, D.C.: American Psychiatric Association, 1985).

11. Robert J. Lifton,. *Thought Reform and the Psychology of Totalism* (New York: W. W. Norton, 1963); Edward Schein, *Coercive Persuasion* (New York: W. W. Norton, 1961).

12. Saul V. Levine, "Life in the Cults," in Galanter, *Cults and New Religious Movements,* pp. 95–107.

13. Larry D. Shinn, *The Dark Lord: Cult Images and the Hare Krishnas in America* (Philadelphia: Westminster Press, 1987).

14. Ted Bohn and Jeremiah S. Gutman, "The Civil Liberties of Religious Minorities," in Galanter, *Cults and New Religious Movements,* pp. 239–253.

15. John G. Clark, "Cults," *Journal of the American Medical Association* 242 (1979): 279–281.

16. Cited in Lawrence Tribe, *American Constitutional Law* (Mineola, N.Y.: Foundation Press, 1978), p. 884.

17. Louis Jolyan West, "Persuasive Techniques in Contemporary Cults: A Public Health Approach," in Galentar, *Cults and New Religious Movements,* pp. 165–192.

18. Shinn, *The Dark Lord,* p. 23.

19. West, "Persuasive Techniques in Contemporary Cults," p. 167.

20. Eileen Barker, *The Making of a Moonie: Choice or Brainwashed?* (London: Basil Blackwell, 1984).

21. Shinn, *The Dark Lord,* p. 133.

22. Galanter, "Cults and New Religious Movements," in Galanter, *Cults and New Religious Movements,* p. 30.

23. J. Thomas Ungerleider and David K. Wellisch, "Deprogramming (Involuntary Departure), Coercion, and Cults," in Galanter, *Cults and New Religious Movements,* p. 249.

24. Brock K. Kilbourne, "Psychotherapeutic Implications of New Religious Affiliation," in Galanter, *Cults and New Religious Movements,* p. 138.

25. Brock K. Kilbourne and James T. Richardson, "Psychotherapy and New Religious Movements," *American Psychology* 38 (1984): 127-144.

26. Cited from the *New Republic* (March 6, 1976) in John T. Biermans, *The Odyssey of New Religions Today* (Lewiston, N.Y.: Edwin Mellon Press, 1988).

27. Richardson, "Negative Religious Bias in the DSM-III and DSM-III-R."

28. Lowell D. Streiker, "Brainwashed or Converted? *The Christian Century* 106 (1989): 722.

29. Levine, "Life in the Cults," p. 106.

30. Paul C. Mohl, "Civil Liberties, Cults, and New Religious Movements: The Psychiatrist's Role," in Galanter, ed., *Cults and New Religious Movements*, p. 16.

31. Franklin H. Littell, "Religious Freedom in Contemporary America," *Journal of Church and State* 31 (1989): 226.

32. Ibid., p. 228.

33. David Bromley and Anson Shupe, *Strange Gods* (Boston: Beacon Press, 1981).

34. Carlton Sherwood, *Inquisition* (Washington, D.C.: Regnery Gateway, 1991), p. 451.

35. Ibid.

36. Lee Coleman, *Psychiatry the Faithbreaker: How Psychiatry Is Promoting Bigotry in America* (Sacramento: Printing Dynamics, 1982), pp. 1, 4.

37. Ibid., p. 5.

38. Ibid., p. 12.

39. Ibid., p. 18.

40. Ibid., p. 20.

41. Bernard Spilka, Ralph Wood, Jr., and Richard L. Gorsuch, *The Psychology of Religion: An Empirical Approach* (New York: Macmillan, 1985), pp. 220, 221.

42. Anson P. Stokes and Leo Pfeffer, *Church and State in the United States* (New York: Harper and Row, 1964), p. 226.

43. E. Fuller Torrey, *Witchdoctors and Psychiatrists: The Common Roots of Psychotherapy and Its Future* (New York: Harper and Row, 1986).

44. Robert J. Lifton, *The Future of Immortality and Other Essays for a Nuclear Age* (New York: Basic Books, 1987), pp. 210, 217.

45. Ibid., p. 219.

5

American Culture and Good Death

For many Americans, good death no longer means patiently letting nature take its course and possibly enduring an amount of discomfort. A good death is increasingly defined as a direct and voluntary preemptive strike against decline and dependence on others, either through assisted suicide or mercy killing. Freely chosen removal of the sufferer now has wide approval. The states of California (1992) and Washington (1991) have gone as far as to place initiatives for assisted suicide and mercy killing before the public for vote. In both cases the initiatives failed, but not by much. Such initiatives would allow patients who are terminally ill, conscious, and competent to request "aid-in-dying." Their written request would be witnessed by two disinterested persons after two physicians approximate that death would occur within six months. The mercy killing would be carried out by a licensed physician through lethal injection. One poll indicated that 61 percent of the populace in the state of Washington supported this policy, and observers are still analyzing the reason for failure. Such initiatives are not without precedents. In Ohio in 1906, Nebraska in 1937, and New York in 1939, legislative initiatives to permit euthanasia were unsuccessful. A physician, Timothy E. Quill, has challenged the medical community with his powerful description of assisting a patient with myelomonocytic leukemia in suicide.[1] A Michigan pathologist, Jack Kevorkian, has assisted a number of individuals with his suicide machine, the "mercitron." In response to Kevorkian, Michigan law now forbids assisted suicide.

The classical arguments against suicide were clearly theological. Thomas Aquinas contended that such acts are contrary to nature and that they encourage others to follow suit, but in essence, he relied on the theological maxim that "only God gives life, and only God should take life away." Proponents of mercy killing now draw on Plato and the Stoics to justify their view, as well as on Sir Thomas More and the poet Petrarch, while opponents draw on Hippocrates and Aristotle, Augustine and Aquinas. It is somewhat simplistic to say that the great divide on this issue lies between Jerusalem and Athens, though in general terms this is so.

The obstacle to the progress of the mercy killing movement in Great Britain and America was the abyss of the Nazi eugenics movement and the appalling revelations of medical killing at the Nuremberg Tribunal.[2] Yet now, with Holland and the Royal Dutch Medical Association placing a de facto imprimatur on mercy killing, with the growth of the Hemlock Society (and its political wing, Americans against Human Suffering), with revelations in major medical journals by physicians who have killed their patients, with polls indicating that 50 to 60 percent of Americans approve of administering lethal injections to unconscious terminally ill patients who have indicated this preference by advance directive, times have changed. There may be no compelling secular arguments against this change.

There are a series of objections to assisted suicide and mercy killing. The two I take most seriously are that the general prevention of suicide is compromised and advocacy for hospice development is weakened. With regard to the first objection, even though most proponents insist that assisted suicide and mercy killing should be limited to terminally ill patients for whom death is imminent (the state initiatives define imminent as within six months), the societal approval of suicide in this narrow context will have implications for other human contexts. Derek Humphrey of the Hemlock Society, the author of the best-selling book *Final Exit: The Practicalities of Self-Deliverance and Assisted Suicide for the Dying*, seems to argue for strict limitation of assisted suicide and mercy killing to the dying, but he goes on to condone these acts for those confronting "degenerating old age." In the chapter of his book entitled "Going Together?" Humphrey condones the suicide of a healthy fifty-five-year-old woman who drank poison with her seventy-seven-year-old dying husband. Even with younger couples, Humphrey sees joint suicide as "an option of very last resort." Those with severe spinal cord injuries are also fit candidates for assisted suicide.[3]

Humphrey states that his recommendations do not extend to those who are simply depressed, but he nevertheless extends an invitation to all of us to set aside the "traditional taboo on suicide."[4] The distressed adolescent can now find this invitation in the self-help sections of local bookstores. Although Humphrey may want to limit the compass of suicide, the net message of his writings is that "self-deliverance" makes sense as a response to many of life's challenges and burdens. After all, if it is acceptable for a spouse to commit suicide in response to the loss of a beloved husband or wife, then why is suicide not acceptable for a parent whose child has died, or for all those whose special relations with family or friends have been undone by disease or aging? It is the spillover from the domain of the dying into other areas of human experience that ought to give pause. The issue must be framed in the context of the common good rather than the rights of individuals.

With regard to the second objection, it is contradictory to think that we will continue to develop palliative and comfort measures to remove pain from the dying when assisted suicide or mercy killing becomes the norm. It is cheaper to dispatch the sufferer than to treat the suffering. Humphrey acknowledges that in most cases, palliation can control pain. But, finally, pain or suffering is not so much his concern as is the sheer assertion of the self's control over death. He even argues that many people in the hospice movement approve of assisted suicide and mercy killing: "There has always been a friendly alliance between many hospices in America and Hemlock."[5] This, however, is not true. David Cundiff, a physician working in hospice care, has written a book the title of which summarizes the opinions of most, if not all, of those in the field—*Euthanasia Is Not the Answer: A Hospice Physician's View.*[6] For those who believe, as I do, that hospices should be at the top of the agenda for health care reform, and that too few health care providers have the knowledge and skills to treat pain properly, the movement toward suicide and mercy killing is clearly a rival rather than a friend. In almost all cases, assisted suicide and mercy killing are chiefly alternatives *not* to pain and discomfort but to the pain control and comfort care that some consider undignified.

My preferred response to this movement toward assisted suicide and mercy killing is cultural, rather than philosophical-analytical, a task better left to others. I will comment on the themes of control, loss of care, and the desire to put an end to human suffering. These themes are not unrelated, and they are deeply imbued in the movement toward suicide and mercy killing. From the outset, it should be clear that I presuppose the right of any individual to refuse life-extending interventions while competent or through advance directives such as the living will or the durable power of attorney.

A HISTORICAL PRELUDE

As prelude, it is useful to keep in mind a typology of attitudes toward death presented in 1988 by Richard W. Momeyer in his book *Confronting Death*. First there is *denial,* a persistent unwillingness to consider the reality of our own death, a kind of lying to the self, possible only when those around us maintain the illusion. Critics say denial inhibits communication and results in a life of superficiality. Second comes *acceptance,* as championed by the death awareness movement. Openness about death, death counseling, discontinuance of life-sustaining measures for the terminally ill, and the academic field of death studies, or thanatology, all interweave to form the "mystique of acceptance." Resistance to death gives rise to a third attitude, *rebellion.* This attitude has roots in the notion that the world is an oppressive place, imposing unfair limits on human fulfillment and achievement. Death is evil because it deprives us of further opportunities and gratifying experiences, and it must therefore be assaulted in any way medically possible. Were I to add a type to the list, it would be love of death, the "death wish" articulated by Freud, that we see in the form of death symbols associated with urban gangs and other subcultures. Here death is desired and pursued through high-risk behaviors and wanton conflict.

Death *is* a massive misfortune, an evil of a sort beyond repair. It is fitting to struggle against it. Rebellion against death has its rightful place. There is a historical debate about whether acceptance is fully possible in the cultural absence of religious explanations that bring order and meaning to life's greatest inequity. I hold that religious worldviews have a highly positive function at this transition point from denial to acceptance (albeit not when they encourage the dying to expect a "miracle" and therefore to pursue futile medical interventions). When David Hume, an opponent of all revealed religion, died peacefully in 1776, a debate followed between "the Enlightenment's party of humanity and the party of faith," as Michael Ignatieff writes in his book *The Needs of Strangers.* Some said Hume's atheist serenity was only a pose. Ignatieff comments that although Hume may have vindicated "the human capacity for self-control" in the face of dying, "he tended to rate the capacities of ordinary mortals much lower."[7] James Boswell, inwardly challenged by the death of his friend Hume, thought that upon the hour of death there are spiritual needs, a yearning for certainties and meanings that religion provides. I side with Boswell and will attempt to enhance the case for religion through reference to the *ars moriendi* and, at the end of this chapter, with the insights of Dostoyevsky.

ATTITUDES TOWARD DEATH

Before turning directly to American cultural history, I provide a wider context for the discussion to follow by reviewing briefly the classic account of Western attitudes toward death by the historian Philippe Aries. For its succinctness, I draw on Aries's *Western Attitudes toward Death: From the Middle Ages to the Present.* Obvious criticisms of Aries might be developed; for example, one wonders whether death was ever as "tame" or unemotional as he suggests. Aries may or may not exaggerate the differences between the past and the present, but the disparities that he points to between then and now are nevertheless valid.

Aries begins with the twelfth century, when knights and monks died in the full and often intuited knowledge of death's approach. The dying made ready for death by carrying out a customary ritual recollection of beloved relationships, and by prayerfully recommending family and friends to God. Dying as an art, the *ars moriendi,* included repentance of past sins, and a deep self-awareness. All this occurred in the bed chamber, which now became a public place; both the dying and those in proximity accepted death rather calmly, without very great display of emotion.[8] Aries contrasts the solemn and "tame" death of the medieval period with the "wild" death of modern times: "The old attitude in which death was both familiar and near, evoking no great fear or awe, offers too marked a contrast to ours, where death is so frightful that we dare not utter its name."[9] Even children viewed death calmly, Aries writes, for they too were familiar with both the dying and the idea of their own death.

But beginning with eighteenth-century romanticism, new meanings were attached to death. It was, in a word, "dramatized" and denounced as greedy, claims Aries. A new cult of tombs, ornate cemeteries, and emotional rhetoric pushed aside the older solemnity and routine as people tried to "steal back" the deceased. There was a new passion in those who viewed death: "Emotion shook them, they cried, prayed, gesticulated."[10]

Dying in the absence of certainty about life after death represented too final a break from the deceased; death became a more hopeless and negative event than ever before, and one therefore resented it. As death gained greater sting, it had eventually to be hushed up, as occurred in the late nineteenth century. Both the sick person and those in proximity were to be spared anguish. Aries concludes that the "procedure of hushing-up began."[11]

The stage was set for death's removal from the home to the hospital. The final days of the dying, once calmly familiar to everyone, were now existentially disturbing in ways they once were not. Aries continues: "Between 1930 and 1950 the evolution accelerated markedly. This was due to an important physical phenomenon: the displacement of the site of death. One no longer died at home in the bosom of one's family, but in the hospital, alone." Even those who can never be restored to health go to the hospital for the sole purpose of dying. Aries concludes with a question that a broadly humanistic approach to medical ethics must ask: "And, on the other hand, must we take for granted that it is impossible for our technological cultures ever to regain the naive confidence in Destiny which had for so long been shown by simple men when dying?"[12]

Writing on American attitudes toward death, Charles O. Jackson observes that there has been a "major withdrawal on the part of the living from communion with and commitment to the dying." He contrasts this to seventeenth- and eighteenth-century America, when life was viewed as a pilgrimage to be endured and relinquished without much resistance (there was little effective medicine with which to resist death anyway). The dying were not hidden away, and "to the degree that belief in a future life was accepted, death did not contribute so serious a challenge as it now does to the individual's sense of self."[13]

But in the nineteenth century, Americans came to view death not as a deliverance from the world's sadness, or as a rite of passage to another destiny, but as final loss: "Increasingly," Jackson writes, "death was perceived within a context of attachment to life as well as some disquieting uncertainty about the future of the dead." Death became less acceptable, so "the living demanded that its harsh reality be reduced, muted, and beautified."[14] Hence the corpse, previously deemed unimportant, became precious and worthy of ornate burial containers. In the Civil War period, protective embalming was instituted, and gravestone sculpture appeared. Americans were clinging to corpses and their memories of the dead because death was no longer a solemn transition to immortality and eventual reconciliation but was now disturbingly final.

The advent of Darwinism and materialistic philosophies of the self meant the loss of the soul, explains Jackson, a loss making death onerously final, and too great a burden to be spoken of. He concludes, "In any event, a dimension of the secular vision in America and elsewhere has been that death became a taboo topic."[15] The deceased were now lost in soul as in body.

Solemnity and peace are now difficult to sustain, perhaps because the mystical explanations that undergirded the *ars moriendi* of old are more or less ruled out in our culture, so neither the dying nor the family can easily give a peaceful meaning to death. As David E. Stannard states the problem, "The answers of the past are no longer appropriate; the answers of the present are insufficient."[16]

Even now, after Geoffrey Gorer, Herman Feifel, Elisabeth Kübler-Ross, and others in the death awareness movement have articulated the importance of tame dying in the midst of supportive love, Americans still struggle to relinquish the rebellion against death when rebelliousness becomes futile. There is no good reason to suggest that in an era of technological gain, people should resign prematurely to the shadow of death. Yet because death is feared in ways that it once was not as our understandings of human nature and spiritual destiny have narrowed, the transition from rebellion to acceptance is not easy. Technological dominance does not facilitate this transition.

A decade ago Aries wrote these words in his book entitled *The Hour of Our Death*: "Although it is not always admitted, the hospital has offered families a place where they can hide the unseemly invalid whom neither the world nor they can endure." As Aries continues, our medical technology is frequently what we "offer" the dying, and this gives the hospital a monopoly on death. "By a swift and imperceptible transition," he writes, "someone who was dying came to be treated like someone recovering from major surgery."[17] The importance of religion and theology in making death acceptable lost ground.

Secularization makes acceptance of death more difficult. There are certainly other relevant social factors. Urbanization removes us from nature and a witnessing of the cycle of life and death; nuclear families have replaced extended families, so that the sense of loss over the death of a loved one is intensified;[18] the extension of the average human life span from three decades to seven means that the child will generally not witness deaths of siblings, parents, or friends; and when death occurs, specialists in the funeral business make it unlikely that the family will ever deal with the corpse. In the final analysis, however, denial and rebellion have deep roots in the loss of theological anthropology. Spiritual rites of passage are lost to metallic ones.

MERCY KILLING: CONTROL, CARE, SUFFERING

Mercy killing can be critically interpreted in the light of reflection on control, care, and suffering. I now turn to this reflection, placing mercy killing in further cultural perspective.

Control

Modern technological culture encourages ever greater control over human events. American families often want their loved ones to die in the controlled environment of the medical intensive care unit. The beeping signals and flashing lights of the machine signify a mastery over nature and human nature. For many, these machines define the best standard of care, and any shift away from this perceived standard is downgrading and therefore undesirable. So, frequently, families resent the offer to move a dying patient from intensive care to a special care unit that provides care and comfort only. Americans often think that if they do not avail themselves of the latest technology, they are missing out.

The idea of throwing in the towel, of leaving death in the hands of nature or of a wisdom that underlies nature, is anathema to the rage for control. We witness the same rage in our era of the "perfect" baby, and with the advent of the human genome initiative, selective abortion of all but one's idiosyncratic aesthetic image of a cosmetically ideal child is increasingly possible. Some will want to control everything from hair color to height. Fetal cells in the maternal circulation will provide DNA profiles of the fetus. Researchers want to control the aging process with growth hormone or scavenger cells. From the womb to the tomb, technological control is the cultural mandate. With the *ars moriendi*, it was the dying person's *internal* control over a rite of passage that brought order. This inward control has largely given way to mechanical control.

Death by lethal injection is best understood as a further act of technological control. It is driven by the *will to control*, to remove human events from the domain of nature, even when suffering can be mitigated in almost all cases by proper palliation. Against this form of control there is only the sense that the hour of death is rightly decided by a wisdom beyond us, that life is God's to give and to take away. To return death to the state of nature requires the assumption that underlying nature is the wisdom of God, of some higher purpose or regulation. Ordinary Americans who oppose mercy killing appeal not to philosophical arguments but to straightforwardly theological ones.

The technological control we do need is in pain control. New modalities of palliation that leave the patient in a reasonably clear state of consciousness are emerging. Electrodes implanted into brain or nerve can modulate pain pathways. Through surgical and cryonic neuro-ablation, pain can be managed in remarkable ways. Our approach to pain management must be physical, psychological, multidisciplinary, and spiritual. But in our curative and rescue-oriented health care system, management of pain is *not* a priority.

Ignorance of proper pharmacologic principles is pervasive, and physicians are often ill-equipped. Medical schools do not include pain management in their core curriculum. Narcotics are administered on a pain-contingent basis, rather than on time contingency; we wait for the patient to express pain. This is ethically wrong.

Caring

To a degree, mercy killing is also the result of a culture that devalues caring. Our medical system concentrates on research and training that steals people back from death. It is rescue oriented in the extreme. Daniel Callahan is right when he refers to "the bias toward acute-care, high-technology medicine, with its comfortable presumption that it *does* something for people in contrast to merely holding their hands." Merely caring suggests acting by default. In a highly compassionate call for the recovery of caring, he continues: "At the center of caring should be a commitment never to avert its eyes from, or wash its hands of, someone who is in pain or suffering, who is disabled or incompetent, who is retarded or demented; that is the most fundamental demand made upon us."[19]

One might contest Callahan's idea of rationing life-saving health care based on old age alone, but it must be said that his efforts to bring care "as a positive emotional and supportive response" into symmetry with technological interventions is fully valid. He is appropriately critical of our failure to train medical students to care in the seminal sense of the word, and he is also right in his pessimism that however much care is discussed in glowing terms, "it always loses out to an emphasis on scientific knowledge and technical skills, and there is no end in sight to that bias."[20] Technology has muscled aside the most basic expressions of care.

It was not always so. Once, there was little the nurse or physician could do but hold the dying patient's hand, usually at home and with some religious motivations. Now, we need to recover such simplicity once rebellion against dying becomes futile.

The caring that the dying really need, other than palliative, is a compassionate response, an enduring, supportive emotional intimacy. In a culture where passion is more highly valued than compassion, the tasks of caring are readily viewed as demeaning. Partial or constant dependence on others is viewed as an unreasonable imposition on them and as personally degrading, never mind that receiving care is a basic human need and giving care is a moral good. Mercy killing has an appeal when the forms of caring that make it unnecessary are systematically de-emphasized and devalued.

Suffering

A culture of external, as contrasted with internal, control merges with the loss of caring in the most basic sense of the word. A third ingredient is this: American culture is extreme in its desire to eliminate suffering. It is remarkable, if Aries is right, that in earlier times suffering was accepted as much as appears to have been the case, despite the absence of palliative methods. Now, utilitarians speak of the "greatest happiness of the greatest number," and our advertisements inculcate the notion that to be acceptable and good one must be zestfully happy. Morbidity and the decline of dying are antithetical to the dominant image of human normalcy, for they require us to face our limits. Mercy killing is conceptually flawed if the motive is the elimination of suffering. Human beings always have and always will suffer. The Tantric Buddhist maintains that if you are born, you will suffer; life is understood as suffering unto growth, until the wheel of rebirth is finally escaped. Christianity makes the cross its central symbol. In a culture that can no longer depend on religious recognitions of human finitude, decline and suffering must be removed from the scene.

Will initiatives like the one in Washington State win over American culture? Or will we look for better ways to control pain, explore a wider range of forms of supportive care, and allocate resources so that long-term care does not require spending to the point of poverty? Acts of assisted or unassisted preemptive suicide and mercy killing are one possibility. The other possibility is to understand mercy, not in terms of killing, but in terms of providing care. For all the vast literature on mercy killing, one of the most persuasive pieces remains Arthur Dyck's "Beneficent Euthanasia and Benemortasia: Alternative Views of Mercy."[21] Dyck stresses pain relief by dosages of medicine sufficient to accomplish this purpose; relief of suffering through companionship; a patient's right to refuse treatment; and a health care system that does not impose such financial pressure on patients or their families that mercy killing becomes attractive. He also emphasizes that if our culture so desires, "mercy" can mean loyal, compassionate long-term caring of the dying, rather than merciful killing.

RECOVERING VIRTUE

In this final segment, I want to return to my original historical theme about the good death, the *ars moriendi,* and the recovery of virtue. And since we are, every one of us, slowly dying as we age, I focus on elderly people. The infirmities of old age and the limitations they impose must be frankly acknowledged. Through emphasis on moral and spiritual values, the stages of outward decay can be transformed into opportunities for inward growth. As Thomas R. Cole has emphasized in his studies of aging and American culture, "hope and triumph were linked dialectically to tragedy and death" in the Puritan tradition.[22]

This dialectic is in tension with attempts to abolish the decline of aging through promises of protracted youth, perhaps through biomedical research on the scavenger cells that destroy the "free radicals" partly responsible for biological decline. How can the problem of meaning and biological aging be faced when myths are prevalent about progressive bio-medical abolition of growing old, and now about the promise of cryonic brain storage with the hope of eventual immortality? Daniel Callahan rightly points out that medical advance, or the endless promises thereof, "reshapes our notion of what it is to live life," dismantling "the cultural attitudes and institutions designed to live within those barriers."[23] Or as Cole suggests, "Unable to infuse decay, dependency, and death with moral and spiritual significance, our culture dreams of abolishing biological aging."[24]

In the modern West, old age is often viewed as a period of consumption in a "golden age" of vibrancy and energy, as though decline can be avoided. We now see books such as Robin N. Henig's *The Myth of Senility.*[25] By contrast, a more meaningful and realistic view consistent with the facts of human decay and mortality emerges from traditions that stress moral and spiritual growth. In the past, the meanings discovered in growing old were embedded in religious worldviews that valued resignation, self-transcendence, and the virtuous life.[26] Harry R. Moody describes the more traditional worldview thus: "In this view, the elderly are not held to be morally superior but rather further along on a journey of life, with life seen as a movement of lifelong fulfillment whose consummation is found only in death and afterlife. The sufferings of old age, in the traditional view, are seen against the wider background of the cosmos. The loss of that wider perspective is partly what deprives aging of meaning."[27] Aging is best understood, Moody contends, as a valued movement under a sacred canopy, consistent with religious meanings that inform life in all its stages.

The eminent historian of American Methodism, E. Brooks Holifield, writes that throughout the early nineteenth century, "Methodists retained the dual sense of death as both penalty and promise." Methodist devotional writings urged the believer to be always mindful of death, since the Christian "lives for death," and should manifest a "joyful, heavenly, and serene" countenance grounded in the knowledge that through Christ "the sting of death was plucked out."[28]

In conclusion, I present a literary example of the good death as I view it. Dostoyevsky published *The Adolescent (or A Raw Youth)* in 1874. The reception was unfriendly, and the book is not one of the author's best known. Yet as a study on death and growing old, it is a classic. In *The Adolescent*, Makar Ivanovich Dolgoruky is a former serf, now old and gray, and the legal husband of "the adolescent's" mother. "The adolescent," Arkady Dolgoruky, narrates his dialogue with Makar, who offers this description of virtuous dying: "So a pious old man must be content at all times and must die in the full light of understanding, blissfully and gracefully, satisfied with the days that have been given him to live, yearning for his last hour, and rejoicing when he is gathered like a stalk of wheat unto the sheaf when he has fulfilled his mysterious destiny." Arkady notes of Makar that "There was gaiety in his heart and that's why there was beauty in him. Gaiety was a favorite word of his and he often used it."[29] Makar seems to rejoice in the existence of things around him, whether human or nonhuman, animate or inanimate. His appreciation of the mystery of the world moves him far beyond a merely utilitarian relationship with the people and objects he encounters. He does not seek to turn the world to his advantage; he values things and people simply on the basis of their being. Arkady evidently feels this "gaiety" of heart, this mystical love for the world that is so different from mere aesthetics.

Arkady continues: "Moreover, I'm sure I'm not just imagining things if I say that at certain moments he looked at me with a strange, even uncanny love, as his hand came to rest tenderly on top of mine or as he gently patted my shoulder." It is love that is Makar's chief virtue. Speaking of death he comments:

> And grass will grow over his grave in the cemetery, the white stone over him will crumble, and everyone will forget him, including his own descendants, because only very few names remain in people's memory. So that's all right—let them forget! yes, go on, forget me, dear ones, but me, I'll go on loving you even from my grave. I can hear, dear children, your cheerful voices and I can hear your steps on the graves of your fathers; live for some time yet in the sunlight and enjoy yourselves while I pray for you and I'll come to you in your dreams. . . Death doesn't make any difference, for there's love after death too![30]

Arkady observes that Makar likes most to talk about religion, about legends of ascetics from the remote past he had heard "from simple, illiterate folk."

I do not present the material from Dostoyevsky to be sermonic or moralistic in tone. Nor do I claim to present virtue theory in any careful or valuable manner, since it is not my forte. My simple point is that Dostoyevsky illustrates well spiritual growth in love for others reciprocally related to love for God, which comes to the true meaning of death as it does to the true meaning of life. A good death is a virtuous one rather than merely an accepting one; it is a death in *amicitia spiritualis* (spiritual friendship) rather than one solely in Hume's serenity.

NOTES

1. Timothy E. Quill, "Death and Dignity: A Case of Individualized Decision Making," *New England Journal of Medicine* 324 (1991): 691–694.

2. Robert N. Proctor, *Racial Hygiene: Medicine under the Nazis* (Cambridge: Harvard University Press, 1988).

3. Derek Humphrey, *Final Exit: The Practicalities of Self-Deliverance and Assisted Suicide for the Dying* (Eugene, Ore.: Hemlock Society, 1991), pp. 83, 100, 102.

4. Ibid., p. 83.

5. Ibid., p. 35.

6. David Cundiff, *Euthanasia Is Not the Answer: A Hospice Physician's View* (Totowa, N.J.: Humana Press, 1992).

7. Michael Ignatieff, *The Needs of Strangers: An Essay on Privacy, Solidarity, and the Politics of Being Human* (New York: Viking, 1985), pp. 85, 95.

8. Phillippe Aries, *Western Attitudes toward Death: From the Middle Ages to the Present*, trans. Patricia M. Ranum (Baltimore: Johns Hopkins University Press, 1974), p. 12.

9. Ibid., p. 13.

10. Ibid., pp. 56, 59.

11. Ibid., p. 87.

12. Ibid., pp. 87, 107.

13. Charles O. Jackson, ed., *Passing: The Vision of Death in America* (Westport, Conn.: Greenwood Press, 1977), pp. 6, 7.

14. Ibid., p. 61.

15. Ibid., p. 235.

16. David E. Stannard, ed., "Introduction," *Death in America* (Philadelphia: University of Pennsylvania Press, 1975), p. viii.

17. Phillipe Aries, *The Hour of Our Death*, trans. Helen Weaver (New York: Alfred A. Knopf, 1981), pp. 571, 584.

18. Robert Jay Lifton, *Death in Life: Survivors of Hiroshima* (New York: Random House, 1968).

19. Daniel Callahan, *What Kind of Life: The Limits of Medical Progress* (New York: Simon and Schuster, 1990), pp. 144, 145.

20. Ibid., p. 147.

21. Arthur Dyck, "Beneficent Euthanasia and Benemortasia: Alternative Views of Mercy," in Marvin Kohl, ed., *Beneficent Euthanasia* (Buffalo: Prometheus Press, 1975), pp. 117–129.

22. Thomas R. Cole, "The 'Enlightened' View of Aging." *Hastings Center Report* 13, no. 3 (June 1983): 35.

23. Callahan, *What Kind of Life*, p. 25.

24. Cole, "The 'Enlightened' View of Aging," p. 39.

25. Robin M. Henig, *The Myth of Senility: The Truth about the Brain and Aging* (Glenview, Ill.: Scott, Foresman, 1988).

26. Stephen G. Post, "Growing Old: Meaning, Religion, and Wisdom," *Gerontologist* 30 (December 1990): 845–847.

27. Harry R. Moody, "The Meaning of Life and the Meaning of Old Age," in Thomas R. Cole and Sally Gadow, *What Does It Mean to Grow Old?* (Durham, N.C.: Duke University Press, 1986), p. 31.

28. E. Brooks Holifield, *Health and Medicine in the Methodist Tradition: Journey toward Wholeness* (New York: Crossroad, 1986), pp. 90, 91.

29. Fyodor Dostoyevsky, *The Adolescent (or A Raw Youth)*, quoted in Hutterite Brethren, ed., *The Gospel in Dostoyevsky: Selections from His Works* (Ulster, N.Y.: Plough Publishing House, 1988), pp. 219, 229.

30. Ibid., pp. 221, 226, 229.

6

The Covenant of Basic Caring

Care for another is a form of anxiety or solicitude for his or her welfare. It is an abrogation of the self-centered tendency and a transfer of interests to another for his or her own sake, on the basis of the other's positive properties or existence per se. Care responds to the suffering of the other; is steadfast and patient; honors the other's freedom, integrity, and individuality.

The measure of our care is the degree of our anxiety. To care is to be neither indifferent nor unconcerned; something at least does matter and therefore cannot be treated apathetically. The controlling motive must always be the good of others, so selfishness fades. Care is not among the acquisitive tendencies such as desires for food, drink, possessions, and merely instrumental relations with others. A strictly acquisitive love is not caring at all, because it implies indifference to the other's welfare except as a means to self-gratification, that is, as a means of acquiring a good for the self, with benevolence never a controlling motive. For care to be genuinely present, assisting and protecting others must be the controlling motive. Care and indifference to the other's good are incompatible. Good for the self, while not controlling, can acceptably remain as a subsidiary motive, for example, personal satisfaction in caring, moral development, mutuality, or social recognition. Care requires the abrogation of selfishness, but it is a mistake to confuse the valid ideal of unselfishness with selflessness, its invalid exaggeration. Selflessness violates the reciprocal structures of most social existence and obscures the extent to which self-concern or care of the self is necessary for care of another to be sustained in commitment.

Moreover, selflessness is questionable because it invites exploitation of the moral agent and fails to correct the other's harmful behavior.

The current plethora of health-related uses of the term "care" tends to confuse its moral underpinnings. "Care" is used to describe high technology and a health "care" industry. But in fact "care" in its basic sense has to do with the daily-life issues to which nurses often respond. Here "care" is the work of a solicitous person dedicated to maintaining the vital functions and to protecting the life and dignity of another. Sally Gadow, in her article entitled "Covenant without Cure: Letting Go and Holding on in Chronic Illness," distinguished between curing (action directed toward the goal of recovery) and caring (covenantal relationship that is an end in itself). Caring, she argues, is the process of entering another's vulnerability and brokenness.[1] Caring is a matter of faithful solicitude: "As curing is the act of the Promethean hero who steals the fire of life from the hands of the gods, so caring is the act of Sisyphus, forever rolling the rock uphill, only to watch it fall again. While such actions are absurd from a utilitarian perspective, they are filled with meaning if examined in the light of covenant and fidelity.[2]

MEDICAL CARE AS LOVE FOR HUMANITY

Greek antiquity developed the norm of *philanthropia*, or a generous hospitality even to the stranger. One Hippocratic precept is, "Where there is love of humanity there is love of medical science." Influenced by the demands of Stoic ethics, the physician is to assist "even aliens who lack resources."[3] The ideal of love for humanity is found among the Stoics, Cynics, Pythagoreans, Hellenized Jews, and early Christian theologians, where *philanthropia* was often used interchangeably with *agape*, the New Testament Greek word for love of humanity.[4]

The practice of medicine in Christianity was profoundly influenced by the story of the Good Samaritan, who assisted a wounded stranger by the roadside (Luke 10:33–34). Early Christians opened hospitals and made care of the sick an expression of divine care. It is argued that Christianity gave rise to a decisive change in attitude toward the sick, who now assumed an even preferential position.[5]

The story of the Good Samaritan and the requirement that Christians assist the sick disinterestedly (Matthew 25:35–46) deeply shaped Western medical culture. A classic expression of love ethics is that of the seventeenth-century physician Sir Thomas Browne, for whom the foundation of all medical virtue "is love for God, for whom we love our neighbor. For this, I think, is charity, to love God for Himself and our neighbor for God."[6] Women religious in the United States from the Sisters of Charity to the Sisters of Mercy nursed the sick and opened numerous hospitals. During the Civil War and various nineteenth-century epidemics, the actions of these nurses won the respect of American society. Lutheran deaconesses and Episcopalian sisters also engaged in this nursing ministry.[7] A contemporary physician, Edmund D. Pellegrino, writes that the virtue of charity, that is, "benevolent self-effacement" shapes "the whole of medical morals."[8]

An ethics of love or care for humanity underlies much of Western health care. But solicitude for the patient is unfortunately sometimes delegated to nurses or those other than the physician. The pressure of countless technological procedures can even dominate primary care specialties. Technology is important, and given the choice, presumably most patients would prefer an uncaring but technically proficient physician to a caring but mistake-prone one. But the good physician is caring in the most basic sense of the word, listening attentively and with compassion to the voice of the patient. Although our society is increasingly secular, it is important to reassert the role of caring in medicine, even if stripped of theological garb. Nel Noddings views parental affection as the wellspring of all human caring and moral behavior. "The caring attitude that lies at the heart of all ethical behavior is universal," she argues. Noddings does not think that the starting point for ethics should be an analysis of moral judgment and moral reasoning, but rather "our earliest memories of being cared for."[9]

FAMILIAL CARING

Partly because of the miracles of medical progress, many of us live longer and experience chronic illnesses that leave us dependent on others. New-born babies who would have died at birth are now rescued by technology, but often with a quality of life that many would consider unacceptable and that creates huge demands on care givers.

If ours is a time when moral idealism and self-sacrifice for the good of others has to some extent waned, then the recovery of care is important. This recovery can genuinely occur in those familial ties that frequently draw on our moral resources most strongly. But calls for loyal care giving and self-denial in the family often amount to an exploitation of women, and in a gendered society such calls must be met with a certain suspicion. Susan Moller Okin refers to "equal sharing between the sexes of family responsibilities" as the "great revolution that has not happened."[10] She makes a persuasive case for the *equal* sharing of directly caring roles by men and women and for an end to gendered family institutions, that is, "deeply entrenched institutionalization of sexual difference" with respect to familial and social-professional roles. It is absolutely morally unacceptable to encourage family care giving and self-denial without strongly asserting that direct care giving must be as much the domain of men as of women. To be concrete about the burdens of caring, I shape this chapter around cases of illness that stretch care givers to the limit.

The literature in Christian ethics on the proper balance between love of self and love of other is vast. Garth L. Hallett, building on Catholic thought, provides a precise analysis of the requirements of *agape* respecting love of self and others through a contrast of six rival norms: self-preference, parity, other-preference, self-subordination, self-forgetfulness, and self-denial.[11] His main criticism of contemporary Christian ethics is that it has not developed a clear "preference-rule" to balance "mine and thine," and his criticism of the wider historical tradition is that most thought has focused on the extremes of self-preference and self-denial rather than on the nuanced distinctions betwixt and between. Hallett makes a case for self-subordination as the proper Christian norm. He is thus largely consistent with the emergent Protestant position that self-denial in the absence of the duty to love the self is an inadequate norm, since it encourages manipulation and even abuse. Thus, Gene Outka and Don S. Browning, among others, have strongly affirmed an other-regarding ethic that includes a significant place for love of self.[12]

On the one hand, unselfishness and an other-regarding orientation are essential and laudable in a context of gender justice. Normatively, however, the ideal of selflessness is inconsistent with both the psychological and social structures of human experience and represents an exaggeration of the valid ideal of unselfishness. Rather than revisit the various theological debates about self-love, I prefer here to approach the question of love and self-denial in the concrete context of familial care giving.

So often when a parent suffers from severe dementia, a child is born with serious retardation, or a spouse becomes disabled do we directly confront situations that potentially require degrees of self-denial beyond what we anticipate or are fully prepared for. Advances in medical technology have raised new questions concerning the nature and limits of caretaking obligations within the family, for despite the myth that technology relieves us of burdens and permits greater leisure, the reality in the area of health care is quite the opposite. Persons who in a previous age would not have survived illness now continue in ever-increasing dependence, and the families of people with impairment or long-term illness are frequently called upon to serve as caretakers in situations demanding considerably more self-sacrifice than was required of earlier generations.

Of course, it has *always* been the case that loved ones fall ill and become more dependent than we might have anticipated; that situation is anything but new. Yet clearly more people now live into very old age and fall victim to its frailties such as progressive dementia; the filial love of adult children who provide direct caring is thus more widely challenged. There have always been some children born with disabilities, but now we commonly attempt to save them through medical heroics and place them in the hands of parents who too frequently cannot afford to care for them. It is not that in the past people never had their love severely tested, but this testing is now more widespread.

Many of us know of lives that have been profoundly altered by the giving of care to elderly ill parents, children with serious impairments, or spouses with chronic illnesses both physical and mental who will never regain independence. More and more, obligations arise that family members never seriously imagined as real possibilities. The modern nuclear family, now only several centuries old and consisting of parents and children living as an isolated unit, perhaps with grandparents in the home or nearby, faces a caretaking crisis. Single-parent families as well as "blended" families of husband and wife with children from previous marriages must grapple with the question of what seriously ill family members are due and why.

Although the difficult requirements of caretaking must be acknowledged, a case can be made for an ethic of stewardship in the family—an ethic of loyal self-giving that refuses to view others as mere means to our own ends. Several criticisms apply to the work of current authors who, in the light of the considerable inconvenience that stewardship now can create, appear to underestimate the creative fidelities possible within families. Additionally, public policy must recognize that care givers themselves need to be cared for. All too often, public policy focuses only on those individuals in need after their families have found it necessary to relinquish care. Last, the technological expansion of care may well require a religiously based ethic that views caretaking as a praiseworthy and sacred vocation rather than as a hindrance to personal freedom. In this discussion these propositions and viewpoints will be developed in the contexts of conjugal, parental, and filial loves.

Conjugal Caring

Care for a chronically ill and dependent husband or wife can rarely be sustained if it relies on a love that is superficial, essentially self-interested, and lacking in steadfastness. No mere love of appraisal, with its property-based core, can easily last in the face of severe mental illness. Love requires commitment and fidelity, virtues inconsistent with egocentric motives. Theologian James M. Gustafson rightly shows little sympathy for the "egocentric, hedonistic interpretation of the ends of marriage and family," which centers on the ethic of individual self-realization, making self-sacrifice a contradiction in terms. He prefers the image of marriage and family in which we are "stewards, deputies, or custodians of one another and of life itself." For the steward, self-denial is a moral necessity for common life, entailing a "readiness to serve others at inconvenience to one's own interests."[13] The man or woman who quests ceaselessly for wider and more varied experiences, so that all relationships become mere experiments to be abandoned in favor of new explorations, can hardly grapple with the level of commitment that human contingency and vulnerability require.[14]

Some, perhaps many, fear that the technological expansion of care locks them into a life of irrevocable self-denial. When a spouse who in a previous age would have died now lives on for years in a condition of total dependence, perhaps with a form of irreversible dementia such as Alzheimer's disease, a husband or wife is confronted with tremendous challenges.[15] It may be that a purely secular perspective is inadequate to sustain fidelity in such cases; perhaps the mystery of God's own fidelity must serve as the paradigm to be mirrored in our own lives. Stewardship implies a free act of self-giving, which may require a religious framework. The Jewish notion of *hesed*, or steadfast divine love in faithful covenant, and the New Testament injunction of love enjoin an ideal of loyal caring.

The direction in which the notion of conjugal stewardship points is well illustrated by the French existentialist and Catholic philosopher of love Gabriel Marcel. Marcel reacted against Jean-Paul Sartre's assumption that every human being is the enemy of the other, which interprets all human encounters as forms of conflict. For Sartre, freedom and fidelity are opposed: freedom of self demands an individualism unhampered by bonds of love and promise. Marcel prefers the ideals of mutual self-giving and faithfulness to others; he rejects self-enclosed individualism for an authentic existence of commitment to others.[16] "Creative fidelity," argues Marcel, satisfies human longings for certainty and steadfast love; it liberates persons from chaos and unpredictability. A model of conjugal fidelity, Marcel cared for his fatally ill wife for a period of years.

Yet the technological expansion of care threatens conjugal fidelity. Increasingly, to be a steward is to be penalized, for care requires ever more demanding acts of self-denial. As Robert Bellah has pointed out, within American culture, many marry with such values in mind as full communication and self-expression, both of which are essentially incompatible with self-denial.[17] Such values can never sustain the moral duties toward which modern medical technology is driving us in numerous instances, that is, greater long-term dependency on the care of others. A religiously grounded image of marriage, however, insists on stewardship as a vocation for men as much as for women to be supported and sustained in community. Given the technological developments that have altered the biological and moral balance of earlier times, this religious framework may provide hope.

Parental Morality and Imperiled Newborns

The question of what parents owe newborns with serious impairments has recently been so thoroughly discussed that it requires little additional comment. Clearly the developments in neonatal medicine confront parents with dilemmas and pressures altogether unheard of just two decades ago. Now, large numbers of infants with disabilities are brought home from neonatal intensive care units by parents who have almost no public entitlements to support them in the permanent duties they have sometimes willingly assumed, or perhaps have had imposed on them by an overly aggressive use of medical technology. This absence of support is particularly unjust when medical technology is used in the face of the parents' wishes to the contrary. Social workers report "chronic sorrow" on the part of many parents unable to transcend their sense of helpless despair not only because their child is not what they had hoped for but because the economic burdens for the future are so onerous.[18] Moreover, there is strong evidence that divorce rates are high in the families of these newborns because of "burnout," loss of free time, and fatigue.[19] Helen Featherstone, the mother of a son with severe impairments, has written about parental response to caring in these circumstances. Normal children, she notes, exact heavy commitment, but the demands taper off as the children grow independent. Impairment can retard or even prevent this tapering process, "extending a child's dependence beyond a parent's natural strength." "A disabled child," she concludes, often "forces parents to think of their old age in ugly dismal terms." Featherstone cites one mother's response to the burden of care as an example: "And when I project, all I see is a sleepy life of never-ending diaper changing for all of us."[20] Some parents resent the technological expansion of care and understandably long for a less aggressive form of medicine that is willing to let nature take its course.

Yet other commentators describe the ways in which families benefit from caring for a child with severe impairments. Rosalyn Darling, for instance, focuses on the stages of parental adjustment to these children. At first, she observes, parents feel helpless and depressed in the midst of what appears to be an overwhelming tragedy. With support from family and friends, however, this first stage can be quite brief. Then parents can go on to accept their child, especially if support services are available. Parents enter an "advocacy stage" in which they challenge the social prejudices against children with disabilities. Parents and families "in most cases" seem to adjust to the difficulties. For the most part, in the absence of serious personal or financial difficulties, the presence of the child "seems to draw family members closer together as an in group facing the hostilities of the outside world."[21]

The significance of Darling's work is this: if families are given the emotional and community service support required, stewardship can be a fulfilling experience. Stewardship in the light of neonatal advances is always going to be challenging, however, and should not be overly idealized by those who extol the meaning and unity that some families discover in acts of caring. Nevertheless, the work of stewardship can be viewed as a creative vocation, and it is in this direction that agapic thought must press. As Gustafson comments in his argument that parents should care for a child with Down's syndrome, "Finally, my view, grounded ultimately in religious convictions as well as moral beliefs, is that to be human is to have a vocation, a calling, and the calling of each of us is 'to be for others' at least as much as 'to be for ourselves.'" Such a calling does not solve all the complex problems of family caretaking, but "it shapes a bias, gives a weight, toward the well-being of the other against inconvenience or cost to oneself."[22]

Filial Caring

As the proportion of elderly citizens in Western societies grows larger, adult children are increasingly bound by obligations to elderly ill parents. The human life span has been lengthened, leaving many elderly parents in a condition of relative dependence on their adult children.

The philosopher Jane English may too narrowly attach filial obligations to current mutual love. "What do grown children owe their parents?
I will contend that the answer is 'nothing.'"[23] English grants that children
may want to assist parents if a close bond of love and friendship exists, but
this position places filial caretaking on the fragile basis of "spontaneous
love." This raises the question of whether her definition of love as a spontaneous phenomenon is adequate, since Christian thought generally
thinks of love as requiring significant degrees of loyalty and as relatively
steadfast despite times when spontaneity is absent.

I am driven back to the ordinary person who attests to commitments
in the sphere of filial morality, generally based on commitment grounded
in at least the memory of love. Everett W. Hall, the philosopher of "common sense realism," wrote that our knowledge of values must "find its test
in the main forms of everyday thought about everyday matters in so far as
these reveal commitment in some tacit way to a view or perhaps several
views about how the world is made up, about its basic 'dimensions.'"[24] By
and large, then, the Western heritage of ethical ideas has underscored the
importance of caring for the elderly parent, despite inconvenience. Gratitude for parental love and respect for the aging parent as a fully dignified
human being are deeply inscribed in the tradition. Not all the philosophers are ready to jettison the concept of loving stewardship for the aging
parent. Christina Hoff Sommers, most notably, has recently written on
filial morality in a manner consistent with religious tradition. Sommers
warns against the consequences of the modern hostility to the moral practices and institutions "that define the traditional ties binding the members
of a family or community." Before this century, she notes, "there was no
question that a filial relationship defined a natural obligation."[25]

In an aging society, many adult children of elderly ill parents are faced
with caretaking responsibilities of unprecedented magnitude. Feminists
writing on the aging society rightly caution against having too much of
the caretaking burden fall on women, who are already in a "superwoman
squeeze" between job, parents, children, and spouse.[26] Certainly filial love
applies to men as well as women; it is clearly unjust to place unequal burden on women. Given the proportions of the demographic transition to
an aging society, we may well be at the crossroads between stewardship
and the disregard of the aged. Despite the serious pressures of technologi-

cally expanded care, the tradition of stewardship and filial love needs to be sustained. Without this tradition, moral chaos may emerge. Of course for those whose parents have never been loving, and perhaps abusive of their children, filial love and related obligations would not be expected to hold.

THE LIMITS OF CARE GIVERS

These affirmations of self-giving love should not obscure the fact that care givers also need to be cared for. The self that is shattered by coercive abnegations of personal interests, needs, and significant desires will not be able to sustain other-regarding activities for long, if at all. All people have legitimate bodily, psychological, and spiritual self-concerns that accompany their readiness to serve others.

Each of us knows persons who, when confronted with the responsibilities of caring for a chronically ill child, spouse, or parent, have made tremendous sacrifices. Are there reasonable limits to the caretaking responsibilities in such cases? Of course there are power struggles within families that lead the elderly ill to choose a life with persons other than family members—a choice some spouses and mature children might make as well. But is there any moral justification for a family's relinquishing care of a member who desires the love and commitment that a family, at least ideally, can offer? Does stewardship require radical self-denial, or does it require balance between being for others and being for ourselves? Can a care giver make valid appeals to integrity of self and proper self-love? Feminists have rightly pointed out that a crucial problem for women has been selflessness and self-abnegation rather than an inordinate love of self. It is not unusual for women to express the fear that the technological expansion of care will mean for them more oppressive bondage to what has commonly been termed their "experience of nothingness"— the surrendering of their individual concerns in order to serve the immediate needs of others to the extent that they do not have the opportunity to develop as independent persons.[27]

These concerns are valid. It is widely accepted that a concern for one's own well-being is a prerequisite for the self-giving that stewardship demands. Though selfless giving is often idealized, the reality is that those who care must themselves be cared for if depletion and the burnout of

which the literature speaks is to be avoided. Some individuals may be able
to thrive and prosper in the role of steward even if radical self-sacrifice is
needed. Saints and heroes, however, are rare. Thus society must acknowledge that appeals made in the language of "obligation of self" have moral
validity and that stewards can justly call for public assistance in the form
of respite, counseling, and group support.

This realistic assessment of stewardship inevitably leads us to public
policy. One erroneous policy position seems to ignore the needs of family
care givers: "If families would take care of the very young, the very old,
the sick, the mentally ill, there would be less need for day care, hospitals,
and Social Security and public resources and agencies."[28] The good family, we are told, is essentially independent and self-sufficient. It is important that an appeal for familial care giving not be interpreted as an
alternative to necessary public support. In fact, the long-term care now
required demands a policy of emotional and material support for families
involved in the caretaking process. Too much public policy at present
focuses on the needs of the individual whose family has relinquished care
because of a lack of social and financial support. In fact, as Rosalyn Darling insists, society ought not to allow families to become exhausted in the
first place.

Even with an adequate public policy, however, one wonders if the
challenges of home care can be met without community-wide realization
of the vocation of stewardship. At present, there are few areas in the
United States in which the family caretaker receives his or her due.
Among social service professionals a wide consensus exists that the ill and
disabled are more likely to achieve their potential in family, or familylike,
settings; but the family itself must not be viewed as an isolated unit.
Given the frequent absence of support, we must be tolerant of those who
are unable to handle the stress of stewardship and therefore must relinquish direct care. Some philosophers have argued that "ought implies
can," that no person is morally obligated to do anything he or she could
not have succeeded in doing however strong the motivation. It is a maxim
of moral philosophy and common sense that no one is bound to do the
(practically) impossible. Accordingly, no person is morally reprehensible
for having failed to do something that became virtually impossible, no
matter how strong his or her character. Such language does not take us too

far, however, because "can" is always a matter of degree. Clearly it is tragic that family members who want to care cannot do so because of the myth that the American family, like the American individual, must be utterly independent and self-reliant.[29]

The problem of care givers left uncared for is a major one, calling for a redirection in public policy. With scarce support services, families providing home care also face the difficult problem of "competing obligations." The needs of one family member can, in conditions of scarcity, compete so seriously with those of another that the caretaker must relinquish some responsibility. Can there be a moral ordering of responsibilities? Would care for children take priority over care for the elderly because the young have had less opportunity to explore their potentials? If choices must be made, does one care first for one's children, then one's spouse, one's parents, and finally one's siblings? These questions are very difficult and even distasteful; moreover, I know of no moral theologian or philosopher who has attempted an ordering of family responsibilities. In an aging society, and in a technological culture that can prolong the lives of infants and others who not long ago would have passed away according to a more "natural" science, stewardship becomes more complicated; choices may have to be made concerning who can be cared for. I make no attempt here to develop a moral calculus or ordering of family responsibilities, and it may not be a good idea for anyone to do so. We must *not* be overly rigid in this area of ethics, since a great deal of individual heterogeneity in priorities and interpersonal proximities is inevitable. The ordering issue must nevertheless, in the light of the technological expansion of care, be considered by individual consciences.

In some cases, caretaking in the family might be limited on the basis of "release by the promisee." As theologian Margaret A. Farley has written, "Because the obligation to keep a commitment comes from yielding to someone a claim over me, it follows that if the claim is waived or relinquished by the recipient, my obligation ceases."[30] Adult family members might freely decide to forgo treatments that would seriously strain their families. In such a case one has not failed in one's obligation to a spouse or parent; rather, the obligation has been waived.

Long-term caring requires a compassionate response to those who need help with routine activities of daily living like eating, toileting, bathing, dressing, and getting in and out of bed. Long-term caring can require sophisticated medical technologies as well, so that it is increasingly "heavier care than ever before."[31] Caring requires protection of both the life *and* dignity of another. It also requires *enduring* supportive emotional intimacy and encouragement.

I am concerned that care giving as a vocation has been devalued in our society, and even within the family. The tasks of long-term caring are readily viewed as demeaning. Partial or constant dependence on others is interpreted as an unreasonable and burdensome imposition. In my view, caring is a basic human need that reminds us of a fundamental reality: we are human beings who are interdependent. In our age of emphasis on autonomy, rights, and freedoms, it is essential to recognize our inherent dependence on others and the reality of human fragility. At the same time, caring often compels advocacy for the autonomy and rights of dependent people.

The lack of support for care giving is a measure of its devaluation. To do for others what they cannot do for themselves requires, in addition to compassion, great commitment and expenditure of time and resources. But it has been noted that "as a society, we have created a situation in which we place a higher value on the act of flipping a hamburger than on the act of caring for chronically disabled individuals."[32]

Family care givers in need of training, encouragement, and assistance must frequently go to unusual lengths to locate people in the community who are willing to devote their time and energies to assist with the daily tasks of the care giver. We neither adequately train nor adequately compensate care givers; this remarkable omission can blight the lives of vulnerable citizens.

Society must recognize limits to care giving for most people. Before the point of burnout is reached, it becomes the responsibility of society to provide aid. Family care giving is a precious moral resource, and for this very reason it merits careful protection. The surest way to weaken and destroy this resource is to overwhelm it.

Precise limits depend on individual circumstances, and those limits vary. But there is no need to argue about, or wait for, the precise point at which the burden of caring becomes unsustainable. Rather, we must recognize the proportions of the problem, and create programs to mitigate it.

If many intact families provide care that is uniquely beneficial to the recipient, then it is ethically unsound and poor public policy to press them to the point of exhaustion where they will in desperation surrender their parent, spouse, or child to an institution. Everyone loses.

THE STRESS OF CARING FOR THOSE WITH DEMENTIA

Family care givers encounter particular difficulties caring for those with serious behavioral problems. Care givers sometimes put tremendous pressure on the psychiatrist to "do something" quickly about behavior that is offensive or frightening and thus results in emotional strain. Our society has come to expect prompt control of such behavior, often through chemical means. Care givers might already be "women-in-the-middle," dealing with various competing obligations, and an aging parent in a delusional or agitated state is the straw that breaks the camel's back. For these and other reasons, some of them economic, it is difficult to sustain the commitment to methods that are not destructive of whatever rational reflection remains for the patient with dementia. Interventions that do not affect the personal identity of patients insofar as it still exists, which are physically less intrusive with respect to the brain, and which require over time active patient participation both cognitively and affectively are certainly costly.[33]

Although there can be no absolute guidelines in this area, it is clear that technological shortcuts can make the demented elderly passive rather than active agents to change. Society and families know that the human brain is the center of mentation, emotion, and personality, and that ideally speaking, this ultimate perimeter of personhood should not be invaded except as a matter of last resort after less invasive measures have been exhausted. But this ideal forms a dialectic with the realities of cost containment and the stress on the family care giver. There is reason to worry about excessive use of drugs and electroconvulsive therapy in geriatric psychiatry, for our society lives by the quick fix and can easily make scapegoats of the elderly.

Elderly persons, in their inevitable decline, eventually withdraw from some of the interests and pleasures of youth. Whether elderly persons feel more isolated than other age groups is a matter of some debate.[34] There are, however, often cases in which an elderly person suffers from what

Emil Durkheim first called anomie, and what sociologists define as "the homelessness of modernity." Isolation, poor communication, removal from preferred environment, and loss of mobility are problems that can frequently be solved through social rather than chemical means. Yet the basic forms of assistance that such solutions require take resources and a willingness to care in the most basic sense of the term. It is unfortunate that chemical custodianship is sometimes the only timely response.

With specific reference to Alzheimer's disease and associated dementias, Richard J. Martin and Peter J. Whitehouse argue that "behavioral interventions (i.e., making modifications in the environment) are generally preferable to medications for the treatment of most behavioral problems."[35] These authors point out that use of medications is important in cases of depression, psychosis, anxiety, and sleep disturbances. But they urge a cautious use of psychoactive drugs, offering two basic guidelines: first, treatment should be purposeful with the target symptom well defined, and second, as few drugs as possible should be used, starting with low doses, increasing dosages slowly, and monitoring carefully for side effects. Polypharmacy, the use of too many drugs, is a particular problem in this patient population.

Nancy L. Mace suggests caution in using drugs to reduce disturbed behaviors (wandering, restlessness, irritability) "at dosages that interfere with remaining cognitive function and at which side effects occur."[36] She also stresses the importance of changing the physical or psychosocial environment first, prior to use of drugs. James E. Spar and Asenath La Rue emphasize supportive therapy in the early stages of dementia and individual psychotherapy as long as the patient's capacity for insight is preserved. Family intervention is useful at all stages of illness, as are interventions in physical and social environments generally. Various drugs can be beneficial but ought not to be the first recourse.[37]

In the ethics literature, two general value orientations with respect to drugs and mental health are often alluded to: pharmacological Calvinism and psychotropic hedonism. The psychiatrist Gerald Klerman originally drew this distinction. The first view is one of general distrust of all drugs, but especially those that are not clearly therapeutic. It favors verbal insights and self-determination. Psychotropic hedonists, on the other hand, see drugs as the first response to life's unpleasantries.[38] Those holding the first view might deal with a depressed early-onset victim of dementia through psychotherapeutic measures, if possible. Effort is made to engage the patient as an active agent of change, as reasonably cognitively intact and capable of basic insights. Drugs are only a secondary road, less valued than insight and self-determination and not to be resorted to prematurely. By contrast, the psychotropic hedonist is more likely to resort to drugs immediately, since they are a valuable technology.

No doubt, as Ladislav Volicer writes, when behavioral problems include hyperactivity, restlessness, resistiveness, assaultiveness, "many of these problems can be symptomatically managed by modification of the patient's environment, gentle persuasion, and exercise, but in most cases, sooner or later, the patient requires a psychotropic medication."[39] The question is, will recourse to drugs be sooner or later?

There is tremendous pressure to make it sooner. There is the need to control patients in less than ideal surroundings and without adequate care. Concern for pressures on care givers, for example, adult daughters or daughters-in-law, is valid to a degree. Music therapy, art therapy, and group activities for the patient may be unaccessible. It will never be possible to create a state-of-the-art unit for Alzheimer's disease in every nursing home. Unfortunately, the pressure to use drugs for custodial rather than therapeutic reasons, so-called chemical straitjacketing, will remain.

NOTES

1. Sally Gadow, "Covenant without Cure: Letting Go and Holding on in Chronic Illness," in J. Watson and M. A. Ray, eds., *The Ethics of Care and the Ethics of Cure: Synthesis in Chronicity* (New York: National League for Nursing, 1988), pp. 5–14.

2. Richard J. Martin and Stephen G. Post, "Human Dignity, Dementia, and the Moral Basis of Caregiving," in Robert H. Binstock, Stephen G. Post, and Peter J. Whitehouse, eds., *Dementia and Aging: Ethics, Values, and Policy Choices* (Baltimore: Johns Hopkins University Press, 1992), p. 57.

3. Owsei Temkin, *Hippocrates in a World of Pagans and Christians* (Baltimore: Johns Hopkins University Press, 1991), p. 32.

4. John Ferguson, *Moral Value in the Ancient World* (New York: Barnes and Noble, 1959).

5. Henry Sigerist, *Civilization and Disease* (Ithaca: Cornell University Press, 1943).

6. Sir Thomas Browne, *Religio Medici*, ed. F. L. Huntley (New York: Appleton-Century-Crofts, 1966 [original 1642]), p. 98.

7. Ursula Stepsis and Dolores Liptak, eds., *Pioneer Healers: The History of Women Religious in American Health Care* (New York: Crossroad, 1989), p. 6.

8. Edmund D. Pellegrino, "Agape and Ethics: Some Reflections on Medical Morals from a Catholic Christian Perspective," in Edmund D. Pellegrino, ed., *Catholic Perspectives on Medical Morals* (Dordrecht, Holland: Kluwar Academic Press, 1989), p. 277.

9. Nel Noddings, *Caring: A Feminist Approach to Ethics and Moral Education* (Berkeley: University of California Press, 1984), p. 5.

10. Susan Moller Okin, *Justice, Gender, and the Family* (New York: Basic Books, 1989), p. 4.

11. Garth L. Hallett, *Christian Neighbor-Love: An Assessment of Six Rival Versions* (Washington, D.C.: Georgetown University Press, 1989).

12. Gene Outka, *Agape: An Ethical Analysis* (New Haven: Yale University Press, 1972); Don S. Browning, *Religious Thought and the Modern Psychologies* (Philadelphia: Fortress Press, 1987).

13. James M. Gustafson, *Ethics and Theology,* vol. 2 of *Ethics from a Theocentric Perspective* (Chicago: University of Chicago Press, 1984), p. 170.

14. See Robert Jay Lifton, *Boundaries* (New York: Vintage Books, 1970).

15. See Robert H. Binstock, Stephen G. Post, and Peter J. Whitehouse, eds., *Dementia and Aging: Ethics, Values, and Policy Choices* (Baltimore: Johns Hopkins University Press, 1992).

16. Gabriel Marcel, *The Philosophy of Existentialism,* trans. M. Harari (Secaucus, N.J.: Citadel Press, 1956), pp. 74–75.

17. Robert Bellah, Richard Madsen, William M. Sullivan, Ann Swidler, and Steven M. Tipton, *Habits of the Heart: Individualism and Commitment in American Life* (San Francisco: Harper and Row, 1985), chap. 4.

18. J. F. Kennedy, "Maternal Reactions to the Birth of a Defective Baby," *Social Casework* 51 (1970): 98–110.

19. Sandra L. Harris, *Families of the Developmentally Disabled: A Guide to Behavioral Intervention* (New York: Pergamon Press, 1983).

20. Helen Featherstone, *A Difference in the Family: Life with a Disabled Child* (New York: Basic Books, 1980), pp. 19, 35.

21. Rosalyn Darling, *Families against Society* (Beverly Hills, Calif.: Sage Library of Social Research, 1979), p. 172.

22. James M. Gustafson, "Mongolism, Parental Desires, and the Right to Life," in Thomas A. Shannon, ed., *Bioethics* (Ramsey, N.J.: Paulist Press, 1981), pp. 154–55.

23. Jane English, "What Do Grown Children Owe Their Parents?" in Onora O'Neill and William Ruddick, eds., *Having Children: Philosophical and Legal Reflections on Parenthood* (New York: Oxford University Press, 1979), p. 351.

24. Everett W. Hall, *Our Knowledge of Fact and Values* (Chapel Hill: University of North Carolina Press, 1961), p. 6.

25. Christina Hoff Sommers, "Filial Morality," *Journal of Philosophy* 83, no. 8 (August 1986): 439.

26. Stephen G. Post, "Women and Elderly Parents: Moral Controversy in an Aging Society," *Hypatia: A Journal of Feminist Philosophy* 5, no. 1 (Spring 1990): 83–89.

27. The classic theological-ethical statement of this position remains that of Valerie Saiving, "The Human Situation: A Feminine View," in Carol P. Christ and Judith Plaskow, eds., *Womanspirit Rising: A Feminist Reader in Religion* (San Francisco: Harper and Row, 1979), pp. 25–42.

28. Arlene Skolnick and Jerome H. Skolnick, *Family in Transition* (Boston: Little, Brown, 1980), p. 51.

29. This myth is discussed in Kenneth Keniston and the Carnegie Council on Children, *All Our Children: The American Family under Pressure* (New York: Harcourt Brace Jovanovich, 1977).

30. Margaret A. Farley, *Personal Commitments* (San Francisco: Harper and Row, 1986), p. 75.

31. Robert Applebaum and Paul Phillips, "Assuring the Quality of In-Home Care: The 'Other' Challenge for Long-Term Care," *Gerontologist* 30/4 (August 1990): 444.

32. Ibid., p. 448.

33. Gerald Dworkin, "Autonomy and Behavior Control," *Hastings Center Report* 6, no. 1 (1976): 23–28.

34. B. Silverstone and S. Miller, "Isolation in the Aged: Individual Dynamics, Community, and Family Involvement," *Journal of Geriatric Psychiatry* 13, no. 1 (1980): 27–47.

35. Richard J. Martin and Peter J. Whitehouse, "The Clinical Care of Patients with Dementia," in Nancy L. Mace, ed., *Dementia Care: Patient, Family, and Community* (Baltimore: Johns Hopkins University Press, 1990), p. 25.

36. Nancy L. Mace, "The Management of Problem Behaviors," in Mace, ed., *Dementia Care*, 95.

37. James E. Spar and Asenath La Rue, *Geriatric Psychiatry* (Washington, D.C.: American Psychiatric Association Press, 1990), pp. 118–121.

38. Gerald Klerman, "Behavior Control and the Limits of Reform—the Use of New Technologies in Total Institutions," *Hastings Center Report* 5, no. 4 (1975): 40–45.

39. Ladislav Volicer, "Drugs Used in the Treatment of Alzheimer Dementia," in Ladislav Volicer, Kathy J. Fabiszewski, Yvette L. Rheaume, and Kathryn E. Lasch, eds., *Clinical Management of Alzheimer's Disease* (Gaithersburg, Md.: Aspen Publishers, 1988), p. 192.

7

Old-Age-Based Rationing, Dementia, and Quality of Life

In 1984 Samuel H. Preston, a sociologist at the University of Pennsylvania, pointed out that "since the early 1960's the well-being of the elderly has improved greatly whereas that of the young has deteriorated."[1] What has emerged from these and other similar observations is a new adversarial framework for thinking about justice, namely, "intergenerational equity." Elderly people are blamed for the suffering of the young, who struggle with poverty and second-rate educational facilities.

The Gerontological Society of America, in a lengthy report critical of the adversarial interpretation of relations between young and old, acknowledges that the financial and social challenge of caring for the growing numbers of elderly persons is substantial and that inevitably this challenge raises questions about the "quantity and quality of opportunities available to younger generations." But the society also states that the elderly are not all well off, citing data from 1984 that put 21.2 percent of elderly persons (5.6 million) below poverty thresholds of $6,224 for an elderly single individual and $7,853 for an elderly couple. Programs such as Social Security, the report adds, benefit all generations because they relieve the family of providing financial support for the elderly and are thus not one-way flows of resources. The society notes that the trends described by Preston and others "should be very alarming to advocates for the elderly." Elderly persons, the report argues, have a great stake in the well-being of the young, since a vital economy requires a capable work force. Moreover, the elderly have a stake in a government responsive to the needs of all its people, since limited responsiveness to the young suggests that the vulnerable of all ages are in jeopardy. The recommendation of the report is that "those concerned with responding to the challenge of an aging society understand the power of various frameworks to define the terms of the debate, and therefore give careful consideration to the various ways this debate can be framed and to the implications these approaches to policy-making can have for persons of all ages."[2]

Perhaps the most pointed result of the framework of adversity between young and old is the call for categorical age-based cutoffs of life-saving health care. My intent in this chapter is to point out the serious moral ambiguities of age-based rationing, although such cutoffs have a certain appeal because they would immediately solve the growing problem of medical overtreatment of elderly. As an alternative to age-based rationing, I argue for a reasonably "objective" quality-of-life criterion that would categorically prevent any patients with more than mild progressive dementia from receiving other than comfort care. For those who are not demented but who are very old, serious consideration of a responsibility to die inexpensively is appropriate. While I understand the appeal of age-based rationing, in the final analysis I retain a preference for a qualitative and mandatory approach to treatment limitations for those with progressive dementia and a voluntary adherence to inexpensive dying for those who are competent to make decisions.

THE AMBIGUITIES OF OLD-AGE-BASED RATIONING

Categorical rationing of life-saving medical care, perhaps based on a cutoff starting somewhere between ages seventy-five and eighty, would be a serious departure from more individualized modes of care. Proponents must do more than acknowledge that all systems of rationing are inevitably painful for someone. Obviously, some methods of cost containment are less painful than others. Few could be more disruptive of essential social harmonies than age-based systems.

First, age-based rationing threatens to fragment the covenant between young and old, since it builds on an adversarial construct of intergenerational relations. Instead of pursuing justice for all vulnerable people regardless of age, our attention is diverted to a supposed struggle between the generations, as though resources made available to the young must be stripped away from the aged. Respect for elderly people is needlessly threatened as the final stage of their lives becomes dispensable. No policy would more powerfully spell a broken covenant between younger generations and elderly people than categorical age-based rationing.

The fifteenth-century Japanese playwright Zeami Motokiyo wrote a well known No drama about an old crone (a withered elderly woman) who was deserted on Mount Obasute in Shinano province. Several travelers encounter the ghost of the old woman, who had been left to die. "How shameful," she cried out. "Long ago I was abandoned here."[3] Old-age-based rationing proposals are haunted by those who would be abandoned to die.

Second, such rationing weakens the fragile veneer of human equality. As Amitai Etzioni argues, "Like all allocations, bans, or prohibitions based on an irrelevant criterion—be it race, religion, gender, or age—rationing health care to the elderly is clearly discriminatory."[4] Elderly people are segregated into a separate category on the false assumption that they have lived out their best years. Equal regard would then apply only to those under some arbitrary age cutoff. Some proponents of age-based rationing suggest that equality would not be threatened because rationing would apply to everyone, so it is unlike discrimination on the basis of race, religion, and gender. A universal application of a reprehensible practice, however, does not make it just. Age-based rationing is discriminatory and ageist.

Third, such rationing is a threat to human freedom, an essential feature of any common good. Elderly people are heterogeneous, and a just society will respect their reasonable choices regarding medical treatment. Before the individual reaches the point of medical futility, of low probability of success of costly interventions, or of more than mild dementia, he or she should be free to make the decision that life has run its course, that it is time to throw in the towel. To impose an age-based cutoff is to lose ground for personal conscience and reflects an undue pessimism about the ability of older people to make good decisions. I know of no ethical theory so compelling and uncontroversial as to justify, for reasons of so-called justice, the imposition of an obligation to die before one personally thinks that "the flame is no longer worth the candle."[5]

The ethicist Joseph Fletcher, now deceased, provides insight. As an octogenarian, Fletcher refused to embrace age-based rationing because it implied that the old had a "duty to die." Impersonal demographic data were not the criteria upon which Fletcher wanted his life to end. Rather, in a properly individualized manner, he wanted to decide for himself "when the flame is no longer worth the candle, when it's better to be dead, but not for reasons of social justice." Death, he contended, should not be imposed on those who still feel that life is worth living; better to "take comfort in the knowledge that patients and their families, like people in general, are open more and more to giving death a welcome."[6]

Fourth, through age-based rationing, the contributions of elderly people would be lost to society. Many older people have made their greatest contributions to society, family, and friends in old age. Proponents of age-based rationing seem to assume that this extra time is dispensable. But regardless of our culture's cult of youth, human beings are often at their generative best artistically, culturally, and socially in life's final stage.[7] Age-based rationing proposals wrongly assume that the final stage of life is not very valuable, perhaps because it is not often the most economically productive. Certainly the notion that old lives are less worth saving than young ones will not stand the test of cultural diversity.

Fifth, age-based rationing proposals are likely to encourage preemptive suicide among elderly people.[8] No longer allowed access to interventions that may restore them to a reasonable quality of life, they would be condemned to a possibly avoidable and unnecessary downward course that makes assisted suicide or even mercy killing attractive. Abstract theories tend to obscure the brute fact: it is this person who, simply because he or she is old, must face needless relegation to hospicelike care and death.

Sixth, because women outlive men on average, age-based cutoffs immediately raise questions about justice between men and women. It is particularly interesting that the proponents of age-based cutoffs are men. It has been estimated that by the year 2000, there will be 37.2 men for every 100 women who are age eighty-five and older.[9] Thus, the population most affected by age-based rationing is women. To my knowledge, the philosophical proponents of age-based rationing, such as Norman Daniels and Daniel Callahan, have been men who have not given much attention to feminist literature. They are not antifeminist, but they are nonfeminist in their methodology. My own position is that women, who spend so many of their years fulfilling the needs of others through direct care giving, deserve to have their final years of sisterhood or solitude respected as recompense.[10] Nancy S. Jecker points out that because age-based rationing would disproportionately affect women, it is ethically unacceptable.[11]

Rationing health care, if justifiable, should be age neutral. It should limit access to the most costly medical interventions and to ones that may not be so costly but have relatively little likelihood of benefiting the patient. Just where these lines are drawn will vary according to the resources of any particular society, although a reasonably full basic health care package should be available to all.

Limits are easier to accept in principle than in reality. If you or a loved one is denied access to a new chemotherapy because it holds only a 5 percent probability of success, you may well resent the fact that this glimmer of hope, however thin, is not available. Because there is a personal cost to not giving everyone every possible medical intervention when "identifiable lives" are on the line, the idea of rationing costly and marginally successful medical care is challenging. Moreover, it appears to violate the cherished belief that we will do everything possible to save any human life, although this belief can never persist in a time when seemingly infinite medical procedures can be applied to the individual.

The burden rests with advocates of rationing to demonstrate beyond a reasonable doubt that there is just cause for imposing limits, whether in the context of private or public health insurance. It makes no sense to speak of rationing in the absence of scarcity; and it makes no sense to speak of scarcity until fraud, greed, excessive salaries, massive insurance company overhead, excessive profit, unregulated pharmaceutical companies, and laws that encourage defensive medicine or overtreatment of the dying have been largely eliminated from the health care system. Just cause requires that rationing be a matter of final rather than first resort.

Some say that we already ration health care by ability to pay. This wide definition of rationing, however, would cover virtually every aspect of a market economy in which some people can purchase more goods than others, and therefore it seems questionable.

No rationing of health care in the context of private or public insurance should occur without a reasonable consensus forged among those people who will be directly affected regarding both the necessity of rationing and the priorities of access. In Oregon, town meetings were held across the state in order to establish how best to set priorities in health care interventions paid for by Medicaid. The goal was to provide everyone under the poverty line with access to basic health care, funded by savings gained through denying access to the most costly and failure-prone interventions. Critics may be correct in suggesting that those affected by Medicaid rationing were not well represented in the town meetings and that medical professionals ultimately established the priority system. Nevertheless, Oregon must be commended for adhering to the basic principle that active community participation is a necessary prerequisite to any rationing scheme.

Consensus is hard to build. The process must encourage all relevant voices to be heard. Because rationing health care involves nothing less than life or death, imposing a scheme devoid of community understanding and support will not succeed. Ongoing rationing committees, to a significant extent made up of those whose lives will be affected, are essential for acceptance and compliance. Where consensus does not exist, we must struggle to build it.

In the event that rationing health care ever becomes necessary for either the entire population or a portion thereof, it will of necessity be justified on the basis of the common good. So that a basic health care package can be provided to all, some sacrifice of individual expectations regarding especially costly, or futile, or improbably beneficial interventions will be necessary. This might include a willingness to die inexpensively when death is imminent and inevitable, making do with comfort care only rather than struggling to prolong dying at great cost, often in the especially expensive environment of an intensive care unit. A patient might not have access to more costly transplant procedures. Parents might not be able to have an extremely premature infant treated aggressively in a neonatal intensive care unit.

Concern with the common good may come to mean that there cannot be an open-ended right to health care, a right to everything available. A more modest principle may be necessary, such as: "A right to health care based on need means a right to equitable access based on need alone to all *effective care society can reasonably afford.*"[12]

What can society reasonably afford? If just cause for rationing health care is clearly established, it would be necessary to view health care as a fundamental human and social good within the context of other goods. Health care is not the only social good, and it need not take precedence over other essential goods, for example, housing, the war against drugs, education, rebuilding America's industrial base, and restoring our inner cities. It is possible for a culture to become overmedicalized, so that health care pushes aside other equally important goods. If health care rationing becomes necessary, we will need to accept a more modest conception of the role of medicine in our individual and social destinies. A public consensus will be needed to define priorities and to ensure a reasonable level of basic care consistent with cost containment. Such a consensus will have to create a balance between preventive care, rescue medicine, and long-term care. This consensus will be reconstructed regularly according to changing economic realities and technical developments. It already may be deceptive for political leadership to promise universal health care access as though such a right is limitless.

Proponents of age-based rationing should turn their idealism toward measures to curb health care costs that are more respectful of older people, that is, age-neutral rationing that affects people of all ages based on their condition and the cost of life-saving treatment. Age-neutral definitions of medical futility or of poor quality outcome specific to particular disease conditions would be worth considering. But setting limits on the basis of age alone is the wrong approach. As C. Everett Koop warns in the foreword to *Too Old for Health Care?* "I offer one closing admonition: Be careful! Your decisions about someone else's life might affect your own sooner than you think."[13]

SCAPEGOATING THE ELDERLY

Age-based rationing has its roots in criticisms of current policy allowing elderly persons to receive too much of the economic pie through rises in Social Security payments, the post–World War II expansion in pension systems, and the advent of Medicare. The term "welfare for the rich" was coined to designate the portion of Social Security that goes to households with annual incomes greater than $30,000. A typical feature article in a popular magazine, entitled "Grays on the Go," fuels the stereotype that the elderly are all staging one grand retirement party.[14] It is easy to think that in the United States we take from the poor and the young to give to the prosperous elderly.

Reasonable critics will ask why the elderly are exempted from the screenings that other recipients of federal assistance must endure in order to be designated as truly needy. Several decades ago it was mistakenly assumed that all older people were in need of governmental support.[15] This gave rise to public entitlements based on age rather than need. Such a policy may have been necessary at the time, but the economic standing of the elderly has improved over the last two decades, so that some combination of age and need is a better criterion for public assistance. Of course as many as 10 million elderly persons, by some estimates, now remain at or very near the current poverty line. Minorities and women, who generally do not receive much Social Security because they often lack the long history of employment that issues in substantive annual payments into this system, constitute the bulk of the poor elderly. Apart from age, and on a needs-basis alone, a claim could be made that these elderly are deserving.

With one-third of the United States population above the age of sixty, and with those older than eighty-five the fastest growing age group, caring for the truly needy elderly is a heavy burden on the shoulders of society. In 1900, the life span for men was 47 years; for women, 49 years. Now, it is 71.5 years and 78.8 years, respectively.[16] This demographic transition to an aging society is a source for serious concern, and society should not support extravagance on the part of those elderly persons who are in fact prosperous.

Again, though, many of the elderly are not rising at noon only to bask in the sun at the Phoenix country clubs. As Robert H. Binstock warns, the new myth that the elderly are all relatively well-off has "provided the foundation for the emergence of the aged as scapegoat in American society."[17] Poverty among the elderly has certainly not been eliminated. Furthermore, adds Binstock, we must be on guard to prevent any backlash against the elderly in times of economic decline when lack of resources should really be attributed to factors such as the balance of trade and the national debt.

Somewhat paradoxically, through serving the young the elderly help secure their own well-being. In a classic of modern anthropology, Leo W. Simmons examined the moral status of the elderly in primitive societies and found that they are highly regarded where they contribute most to the lives of the young: "Perhaps the simplest and most effective way of eliciting the support of others has been to render essential—if possible, indispensable—services to them." The fact is that the roles of the elderly have in the past "hardly ever been passive" at any stage in the cycle of life. Moreover, their activities have done much to influence their security. Regarding the ancient Hebrews, Simmons writes: "Their security has been more often an achievement than an endowment—an achievement in which favorable opportunities have been matched with active personal accomplishments."[18]

Karl Barth emphasized the importance of the "teaching function" of the elderly, whose insights into traditions both religious and moral give them value in the eyes of the young. And in relation to their own children, writes Barth, "they do not merely represent their own knowledge and experience but that conveyed to them by their own predecessors."[19] In modernity, however, the loss of tradition means that the elderly have limited opportunity to function as teachers; correlatively, the young find no valuable information in what the old convey. It is more difficult for the old to be viewed positively by the young. Ours is, for the most part, a forward-looking culture, and a source of valued knowledge is more likely to be the latest computer software than a wise old man or woman. Still, this is no excuse for ageism and scapegoating.

Rather than categorically relegating people to hospicelike care just because they are old, we might choose to limit treatment for those who have experienced a severe decrease in quality of life. In particular, progressive dementia in its severe stages is an underlying condition that dictates comfort care only, as I will now argue.

PROGRESSIVE DEMENTIA: DISCLOSING DIAGNOSIS

An article entitled "Should Patients with Alzheimer's Disease Be Told Their Diagnosis?" appeared in the *New England Journal of Medicine*. It pointed out that new knowledge about Alzheimer's disease is "likely to swing the pendulum even more decisively in favor of truth-telling." The authors, M. A. Drickamer and M. S. Lachs, refer to new clinical biologic markers that may increase diagnostic accuracy.[20] So long as clinical diagnosis of Alzheimer's disease is uncertain, some clinicians regard it as ethically valid to withhold from patients, even those able to comprehend, information about diagnosis and prognosis. If diagnosis becomes certain rather than probable, this argument will no longer be valid.

Yet is it already invalid? Our's is an era of advance directives, concern with quality of life in severe dementia, and patient interest in controlling decisions about the use of life-sustaining medical interventions in the stages of progressive dementia. Withholding information seems difficult to justify except when a patient manifests clinical depression. The principles of veracity and patient self-determination require that, in nearly all cases, telling the truth to the patient is ethically fitting. Patients have a clear legal and ethical right to decide, while still competent, whether or not they want certain technologies used upon them should they become incompetent. To the contrary, Drickamer and Lachs suggest that this extension of patient autonomy through advance directives may be questionable because (a) the new self with severe dementia is arguably no longer the old self, and (b) the old self may have overly grim views of progressive dementia and fail to appreciate the unanticipated "contentment" of some patients in the severe stages of decline.

Questionable perhaps, but in the final analysis the patient holds the right to make anticipatory choices for the demented self. Respect for autonomy is the moral principle honoring freedom under conditions of competence. Such respect is not an absolute, for autonomy obviously should not be honored above the other strong ethical principles of non-maleficence ("first do no harm") and justice. Other principles, such as beneficence, confidentiality, and veracity, also sometimes come into tension with autonomy. Yet it is well established in ethics and law that autonomy, or patient self-determination, is prima facie binding on the physician, who may refer the patient to another competent care giver if he or she cannot conscientiously carry out the desires of the patient or the patient's surrogates.

There are some physicians and other health care workers, as well as many family members, who fear that telling the truth will cause distress to the patient, that he or she will feel stigmatized, become depressed even to the point of despair, and become more difficult to manage. So it is suggested by some that the best interests of patients dictate nondisclosure. Most health professionals who work closely with demented patients, however, believe that such concerns are unwarranted, that telling the patient the diagnosis only rarely elicits an adverse reaction. Rather, disclosing the diagnosis to the patient allows him or her to participate as far as possible in the development of a plan of action for the future.

There are important reasons to err on the side of disclosing probable diagnosis. Many patients already suspect that they have Alzheimer's disease, even if family members want to "protect" them from knowing. Some patients want to know their diagnosis so that friends and neighbors will understand that they are not being purposely unpleasant when they forget names. The following testimony, taken verbatim from the Greater Cleveland Community Forum on Values and Health Care, is an example of such a case. Testimony was recorded from Ruth C., whose husband, Murray C., is an Alzheimer's patient. She had been wondering for several months how Murray would respond to her suggesting that he be assessed at the Elder Health Clinic for dementia:

> As luck would have it, he said one day "look what's in the paper here, a doctor is speaking about Alzheimer's at the University Hospitals." Well, I can tell you that was from God, as far as I can see. . . . Murray knew there was a problem, and people with Alzheimer's do know there is a problem and everyone in the family tries to hide it from them, and they try to hide it from the family. This goes on in circles, and from the people I have talked to, they have said that if they could just open up and talk freely to each other, let alone to their doctor, that would be a Godsend.

Ruth C. then describes how Murray wanted to know his diagnosis in order to tell the neighbors that when he forgets them, it is not a sign of arrogance or unconcern. Murray gave slow testimony in still-understandable words that he was deeply relieved to be able to name his disease so friends would understand his limits, rather than take offense at him. Far from causing depression, disclosure brought this patient relief. Joseph M. Foley also describes a case in which the patient was relieved to know his diagnosis and prognosis and thus obviate embarrassment and annoyance at forgetfulness.[21]

The content, the timing, and the manner of the telling must be appropriate for each individual patient. For early or mildly affected patients, doubt and fear of the unknown is replaced by a certainty that may be shocking and upsetting at first but is accepted as reality with the passage of time and the establishment of supports. All experienced health care professionals have known families who have agonized about telling the patient about a diagnosis of, for example, Alzheimer's disease, only to have the patient say, "That's what I've thought all along."

Ideally, the physician, the nurse, and the social worker who have participated in the investigation and have developed rapport with patient and family should be present and involved. A specific plan of action for the future must be agreed upon or at least proposed. The patient and the family should be encouraged to ask any questions at all, either at the meeting or in the future. About what the patient should be told, much depends on the patient's ability to understand, but he or she should be told that something is wrong, the situation is not normal; that the problem results from changes in the brain and is not an emotional problem alone; that it is a serious condition, to be taken seriously by the patient, the family, and the physician. In the case of the progressive degenerative dementias like Alzheimer's disease, where the issue of disclosure most often arises, other information should be given: that the causative condition is a known disease of the brain; that the expectations for the future, although uncertain, are in general predictable; that although the disease cannot be cured, its effects can be treated; that the understanding and cooperation of the patient will make things better for everybody; and that the health care team will be available to help all the way.

Patients with dementia have varying degrees and kinds of insight. A widely expressed and very wrong opinion is held that patients with dementia are not aware that they are demented. In fact, there is a wide spectrum of insight. At one end are the patients who even in the early stages have anosognosia for their condition, probably because of the nature of their brain lesions. The failure to be aware in this sense means that the patient is incapable of accepting contrary opinion and tries to behave as if he or she were normal. Another group of patients go through an active denial process, similar to that seen in nondementing organic disease. Still others, aware something is wrong, make usually inept efforts to conceal their feelings. Probably the largest number of patients are aware that they are not normal. If they do not put it in words, their acceptance of dependence points to a preservation of some insight.

QUALITY OF LIFE AND COMFORT CARE ONLY

There is wide debate over the morally appropriate levels of medical care for patients in the advanced stages of progressive and eventually fatal dementia such as Alzheimer's disease. This debate focuses on the definition of "quality of life" and the related ethical question of whether life-extending medical interventions should be used for reasons other than comfort and palliation when quality of life has severely deteriorated.

There are important cautions about using quality of life as an indicator of appropriate treatment levels: quality of life is partly contingent on the extent to which a supportive environment is created to enhance well-being; a fully reliable qualitative measure of a patient's experience is impossible; quality of life has a subjective aspect, so only the person whose life it is can assess quality; and the idea of quality of life can be misused to rid society of unproductive members. Yet, nevertheless, appeal is commonly made to quality of life in clinical discussions with patients regarding treatment limitation, or with patient surrogates.

There are two major quality-of-life thresholds that are often evident in discussion: the loss of the capacity to relate to others, in which neither recognition nor communication is possible; and the probable loss of self-identity, that is, of psychological continuity between past and future. Some physicians may take a less relational view of quality of life, since patients lacking relational capacities can demonstrate underlying affective responses and may retain greater self-awareness than relational incapacities suggest. Quality of life for patients with progressive dementia might be assessed with emphasis on any of the following capacities: to make judgments and solve problems; to remember recent events; to remember past events; to handle business, financial, or social affairs; to pursue hobbies and interests; to form and maintain relationships with others; to recognize close family members or friends; to recognize others generally; to experi-

ence emotions; to recognize oneself; to plan for the future; to eat; to control excretory organs; and to communicate through speech. There are
probably other capacities to be considered as well.

My interest in the opinion of the physician regarding quality of life
and its moral significance, if any, in no way questions the right that people
with dementia or their surrogates have to participate in and to have final
authority in making decisions. The implementation of this right among
the elderly continues to be a topic of considerable empirical investigation.
Yet attention to physician opinion is justified, since most clinical decisions
occur in the context of discussion between doctor and patient or family
surrogates, and in part the values of the physician shape consensus. It is
beneficence, not authoritarianism, that prompted F. J. Ingelfinger to
argue that physicians have an obligation respectfully to recommend a
course of action, rather than simply lay out the alternatives and abandon
patients.[22] The physician as well as the patient has a moral voice, which
calls for an "ethics of communication."[23] The physician must be "a moderate autonomist and a moderate welfarist."[24]

There are several relevant questions for future research. To what
extent does consensus exist among physicians that life-extending interventions should not be used in various levels of severity except for purposes of
comfort and palliation? What is the relationship of physicians' views on
the use of life-extending interventions to their age, gender, medical spe-
cialization, clinical setting, experience with patients suffering from Alzheimer's disease, and experience with a close relative with Alzheimer's
disease?

Within the medical community, "consensus breaks down when the
attempt is made to determine the nature of the therapeutic obligation to
the demented patient, particularly with respect to life-sustaining treatment."[25] L. Volicer detected lack of consensus regarding patients in the
persistent vegetative state, and in advanced dementia.[26] In a 1991 cross-
national empirical study of physicians' attitudes toward life-extending
treatment interventions for elderly people with severe dementia, considerable disagreement was evident. The authors asked, "What decisions
would physicians make when confronted with a critically ill, demented
elderly man?" They presented the case of an eighty-two-year-old man
with life-threatening gastrointestinal bleeding who three years earlier had

been diagnosed by a neurologist as suffering from probable Alzheimer's disease. He could not answer a simple question coherently but seemed to understand some simple commands. His behavior was agitated, he wandered, did not recognize his daughter, and had urinary incontinence. In seven countries, physicians in academic medical centers at family practice, medical, and geriatric rounds were questioned about their views on treatment levels. The authors conclude that there is wide variation of opinion both within and among countries. For example, only 6 percent of Australian physicians recommended treatment in a medical intensive care unit, whereas 32 percent of U.S. physicians did so. Conversely, 21 percent of Australian physicians, as opposed to 3 percent of U.S. physicians, chose supportive care.[27]

The variation that this study found is difficult to interpret. No information is provided regarding the reasons for various opinions, level of training, and availability of technology. Most relevant to the proposed project, the authors made no attempt to vary the severity of dementia in order to identify those points along the continuum of decline thought by physicians to be morally significant. So while the study does indicate a useful direction for empirical research, it is extremely preliminary.

It is noteworthy that several philosophers have recently argued that as dementia progresses in severity, only supportive care is morally fitting. Dan W. Brock asks, "What health care and expenditure of resources on health care is owed on grounds of justice to the severely demented elderly?" Brock concentrates on the effects of dementia such as the erosion of memory and other cognitive functions that "ultimately destroy personal identity." This loss implies, for Brock, that the "severely demented have lost an interest in treatment whose ultimate purpose is to prolong or sustain lives."[28] They retain, however, an interest in comfort, so a painful tumor might be removed for palliative reasons. Daniel Callahan points out that the patient who is severely demented, has, on the one hand, "lost his capacity for reason and usually—but not always—human interaction. On the other hand, there will be no clear ground for believing that the capacity to experience emotions has been lost."[29] Callahan's main point is that "death need not be resisted."

Whether the views of Brock and Callahan suggest an emerging consensus is difficult to determine. Yet discussions have matured regarding the moral justification for medical interventions with respect to quality and quantity of life, and regarding the justice of denying access to "futile" medical interventions.[30] Many physicians do not wish to be required to provide interventions that appear futile.[31] A physician writes that "the family cannot demand that physicians continue to give treatment that is not in the patient's best personal medical interest."[32] The goals of medicine are comfort, palliation, and the restoration of health. Given these goals, it may be difficult to defend aggressive treatment for severely demented persons, regardless of an advance directive that might call for such.

Related to the debate about quality of life and treatment limitation is concern with just access to health care. Communities in seventeen states have initiated dialogues about ways to control medical costs and have joined together to form a national organization called American Health Care Decisions.[33] The expense of life-prolonging interventions in cases of advanced dementia is considerable and will further strain limited resources in the future. The cost of long-term care for a victim of Alzheimer's disease was estimated at $25,000 to $65,000 annually. Costs are paid for by the patient, his or her family, or by Medicaid if the patient is deemed eligible according to state regulations. The cost to a family caring for a patient with Alzheimer's disease at home averaged $18,000 per year.[34] The range of costs is considerably higher today, especially for those who require extensive treatments as home care becomes more technical.

Although more studies are necessary, preliminary data indicate that a considerable majority of elderly nursing home residents would want only comfort care and palliation in the event of advanced Alzheimer's disease and that a minority of such residents desire aggressive life-extending treatments. This study of forty-four alert elderly nursing home residents using case vignettes.[35]

For patients in the advanced stages of progressive and eventually fatal dementia, would it be just to impose categorical limits on the prolongation of life, except as a side effect of palliation and comfort care? Although courts have shied away from using quality of life as the foundation for making treatment decisions, and many rely on a patient's wishes expressed while he or she is competent, is so much deference to patient autonomy consistent with justice and the common good?

Consensus building must focus exclusively on progressive and irreversible cognitive decline in adults who were once mentally intact and legally competent but whose disease is in its advanced stages. Thus, my queries are not applicable to patients with degrees of fixed mental retardation or other cognitive impairments that do not represent a decline from a previous more intact mental state. I consider only the primary degenerative dementias such as Alzheimer's disease that eventuate in death and can therefore be reasonably understood as extended terminal illnesses. I recognize that the progressive nature of dementias such as Alzheimer's toward the profound and ultimately terminal stages puts them in a category distinct from nonprogressive conditions, such as mental retardation. Yet some connections might be drawn between limiting aggressive life-saving interventions for people with the severest levels of mental retardation that preclude any possibility of their achieving a personal relationship with another human being, and limiting such interventions for those with severe dementia. Quality of life has often been suggested as a reason for not aggressively saving neonates whose retardation is likely to be extreme.[36] As early as 1976, Robert Katzman wrote, "In focusing attention on the mortality associated with Alzheimer disease, our goal is not to find a way to prolong the life of severely demented persons."[37] My concern is with the loss of relational capacity and self-identity, both critical determinants of quality of life. Because progressive dementia occurs on a continuum, the dementia becoming more and more severe, there are morally significant thresholds, such as when the patient becomes mute and lacks all capacity to interact with others or when he or she no longer recognizes loved ones. These thresholds will not be reached synchronously, but together represent an objective loss of the potential for interactive relationships. Loved ones will often state that the patient is "no longer there." When the patient arrives at these points, has the meaning and substance of human life deteriorated to the extent that the use of medical technologies for nonpalliative reasons becomes morally questionable? In neonatal intensive care units, infant life is saved in the hope that some capacity for interaction will emerge. In the case of advanced progressive dementia, there is no such hope.

Another view of quality of life might attribute higher value to the inner experiences of the self despite the loss of the capacity to interact or might suggest that more self-identity may still be present in the patient than meets the eye. Patients with severe dementia do demonstrate underlying affective responses, and they may have occasional windows of clarity when some self-identity surfaces. But in the profound and terminal stages, there is no discernible self-identity remaining. It is very unlikely that self-identity is maintained; the appearances of loss cannot be explained as a deterioration in communicative abilities alone. Radical decline in self-identity and the capacity to relate to others are inevitably abstractions from a continuum and a set of thresholds that may not occur simultaneously, but they are useful in describing a general distinction between moderate and advanced dementia.

There is no absolute certainty about how and when deterioration in communication and short-term memory gives way to a loss of internal sense of self-identity. As Aristotle argued, however, some degree of uncertainty is an unavoidable aspect of most good practical reasoning. In the traditions of Western moral casuistry, the basing of moral decisions on rough certainty is accepted on the grounds of highly probable correctness, or "probabilism."

To keep a patient with advanced dementia comfortable requires neither causing death by human hand nor striving for prolongation. I do not advocate active euthanasia chiefly because of the possibilities for abuse and because it confuses the identity of the physician as healer.[38] Four Austrian nursing aides, after all, did kill forty-nine elderly demented residents in a long-term care setting. One aide was quoted by police as saying, "The ones who got on my nerves were dispatched directly to a free bed with the Lord."[39]

Unaware of environment, mute, bedridden, incontinent of bladder and bowel, with unmeasurable intellectual functions, and with death inevitable, comfort care is often all that medicine should offer. Comfort care means palliation only; it excludes artificial nutrition and hydration, dialysis, antibiotics, and all other medical interventions unless necessary for the control of pain and discomfort.

If a goal of medicine is justice in the delivery of care, a community consensus may indicate that in order to provide essential treatments for all, intentional life prolongation is not permitted for those with advanced Alzheimer's disease or associated progressive dementias. The principle of comfort care only should not be imposed on patients who still evidence a degree of relational capacity and self-identity.[40]

It is crucial that care and respect for patients be sustained, no matter how advanced their dementia. This means that comfort care must never be withheld or withdrawn and that mercy killing must be avoided.[41] Patients with severe dementia still command basic respect. Yet it is erroneous to attribute purposeful responses to the patient with advanced dementia when in reality there are only purposeless movements. It is a mistake to think of such patients as persons whose experience is merely "different" from that of more "normal" others. Such error is sometimes heard from care givers for people in the persistent vegetative state. The result can be costly and futile efforts to prolong lives devoid of relational capacity. It is necessary to acknowledge, at some reasonable point, that a person has lost the capacities that make human life meaningful. Death is uniformly the result in patients with a degenerative, progressive, and irreversible dementia.[42]

Comfort care for the severely demented person extends beyond that for designated populations such as impaired infants, accident victims with spinal cord injuries, the mentally disabled, and the frail and impaired elderly to encompass the dying. Hospice care merits emphasis, because it is one of the areas in modern health care in which genuine caring remains the essential ingredient. Death is too often denied in American culture, and futile efforts to rescue the dying from its grasp are costly and can sap resources from basic health care that should be made available to all people.

LONG-TERM CARE

If people with severe progressive dementia are to be denied life-saving interventions, they must not be denied care and comfort. Caring is solicitude. It is present to the extent that anxiety is felt about the well-being of another. Modern rescue medicine has often forgotten care in this most basic and covenantal sense of being with the patient. Care giving as a vocation has been devalued in our society. The tasks of long-term caring are readily viewed as demeaning. Partial or constant dependence on others is interpreted as an unreasonable and burdensome imposition. Yet caring is a basic human need that reminds us of a fundamental reality: we are human beings who share social interdependence. In our age of emphasis on autonomy, rights, and freedoms, it is essential to recognize our inherent dependence on others and the reality of human fragility. At the same time, caring often compels advocacy for the autonomy and rights of dependent people.

The lack of support for care giving is a measure of its devaluation. To do for others what they cannot do for themselves requires, in addition to compassion, great commitment and expenditure of time and resources. But it has been noted that "As a society, we have created a situation in which we place a higher value on the act of flipping a hamburger than on the act of caring for chronically disabled individuals."[43] Given this reality, some people who are attracted to the vocation of caring are unable to sustain a minimally decent standard of living for themselves and thus frequently elect to pursue other career paths. Family care givers in need of training, encouragement, and assistance must frequently go to unusual lengths to locate people in the community who are willing to devote their time and energies to assist with daily care-giver tasks. We neither adequately train nor adequately compensate care givers; this remarkable omission can blight the lives of vulnerable citizens.

Complicating this devaluation is the dramatic rise in need for long-term care in all age groups, sometimes a result of medical progress. Life-saving interventions allow people to survive but may leave them in need of extended or even life-long care. Premature infants may be saved through neonatal intensive care and go on to live reasonably independent lives, but some are permanently impaired and dependent on family members in ways that are frequently unanticipated and for which they are ill-equipped. As our human life span has increased from approximately fifty years at the turn of the century to nearly eighty years now, periods of dependence on care givers extend far beyond what was ordinarily the case a few generations ago. Victims of accidents who sustain severe spinal cord injuries generally survive, and with survival come extensive needs for long-term care.

Until this century there was relatively little that could be done for the ill. One famous painting of doctor and patient depicts a bedside scene in the home with family members visible and some religious symbol of care in the background. The physician could take pulse and temperature, and perhaps prescribe a remedy. But the dominant image is of the physician who holds the patient's hand and listens attentively. Virtually all the great codes of medical ethics from world cultures emphasize that the central task of the healer is compassionate caring. As modern medicine became technologically resourceful, technique began to replace caring, although we still use the word "caring" even when little or no real contact with the patient as a person is made. Even in primary care, diagnostic technology now often pushes aside caring. Facilities for long-term care sometimes look more like an acute intensive care unit than a hospice.

Educators in all areas of health care need to emphasize the caring aspect of healing, and the importance of providing long-term care. Although it is imperative that health care professionals know scientific fact, it is equally imperative that they be caring people who respect the rights of those they serve.

SHARED RESPONSIBILITY

Daughters and daughters-in-law are the ones typically called on to provide emotional support and assistance for those needing long-term care. Over the last few years, national attention has been focused on "women in the middle," on women sandwiched between job and family responsibilities. The extension of the human life span means that "contemporary adult children provide more care and more difficult care to more parents and parents-in-law over much longer periods of time than ever has been the case before."[44] Studies indicate that daughters or daughters-in-law are more than three times as likely as sons to assist an elderly care giver with a disabled spouse, and women outnumber men as the care givers for severely disabled parents by a ratio of four to one. Although results vary somewhat from study to study, about half of these women care givers experience stress in the form of depression, sleeplessness, anger, and emotional exhaustion.[45]

Significant numbers of women are harmed by the social expectation that they embrace care giving as their exclusive duty in life, no matter how severe the threat to their own well-being. In response to this harm, policy-makers, researchers, and male family members must give systematic attention to it.

Despite the often unanticipated and unplanned-for burdens of care giving, more than 80 percent of elderly persons with disabilities are cared for at home by their families. At present, social policy often does little more than cheer these families on. Parents of severely disabled children will sometimes succeed against the odds, but there are many who complain about "extending a child's dependence beyond a parent's natural strength." As one mother writes, "All I see is a sleepy life of never-ending diaper changing for us."[46]

Society should *never* assume that care-giving obligations, capabilities, and capacities within the family are unlimited. There are instances of care givers who have sacrificed themselves out of love for a family member and genuinely feel that they discovered themselves in the process.[47] But more generally, extremes of self-denial ultimately take a severe toll on the care giver, and they place the recipients of care at risk for neglect and abuse.

Society must recognize limits to care giving for most people. It has a responsibility to provide aid before the care giver reaches the point of burnout. It is ethically unsound and poor public policy to press care givers to the point of exhaustion, where they will in desperation surrender their parent, spouse, or child to an institution. Everyone loses. Family care giving is a precious moral resource, and for this very reason, it merits careful protection. The surest way to weaken and destroy this resource is to overwhelm it.

At present, long-term care is underfinanced, especially in comparison to available acute care medical services.[48] Respite care, day care, in-home services, and a broad array of community-based programs could make the burden of care giving more tolerable. A proper balance must be established among preventive, acute, transitory, and long-term care services and facilities.

NOTES

1. Samuel H. Preston, "Children and the Elderly in the U.S.," *Scientific American* 251, no. 6 (1984): 44.

2. Eric R. Kingson, et al., *Ties That Bind: The Interdependence of Generations (A Report of the Gerontological Society of America)* (Washington, D.C.: Seven Locks Press, 1986), pp. 2, 3, 120, 165.

3. Zeami Motokiyo, "The Deserted Crone," in G. L. Anderson, ed., *Masterpieces of the Orient* (New York: W. W. Norton, 1977), p. 715.

4. Amitai Etzioni, "Health Care Rationing: A Critical Evaluation," *Health Affairs* 10, no. 2 (Summer 1991): 94.

5. Joseph Fletcher, "Ethics and Old Age," *Update: Ethics Center of Loma Linda University* 4, no. 1 (1988): p. 4.

6. Ibid.

7. Thomas P. McDonnell, "America's Obsession with Youth—Some Literary Origins," *This World: A Journal of Religion and Public Life* 16 (Winter 1987): 105–109.

8. C. G. Prado, *The Last Choice: Preemptive Suicide in Advanced Age* (New York: Greenwood Press, 1990).

9. Stephen G. Post, "Justice for Elderly People in Jewish and Christian Thought," in Robert H. Binstock and Stephen G. Post, eds., *Too Old for Health Care? Controversies in Medicine, Law, Economics, and Ethics* (Baltimore: Johns Hopkins University Press, 1991), p. 124.

10. See Stephen G. Post, "Women and Elderly Parents: Moral Controversy in an Aging Society," *Hypatia: A Journal of Feminist Philosophy* 5, no. 1 (Spring 1990): 83–89.

11. Nancy S. Jecker, "Age-Based Rationing and Women," *Journal of the American Medical Association* 266 (1991): 3012–3015.

12. Larry R. Churchill, *Rationing Health Care in America: Perceptions and Principles of Justice* (Notre Dame: University of Notre Dame Press, 1987), p. 94.

13. C. Everett Koop, Foreword to Binstock and Post, *Too Old for Health Care?* p. x.

14. N. R. Gibbs, "Grays on the Go," *Time* 131, no. 8 (1988): 66–75.

15. Robert H. Binstock, "The Aged as Scapegoat," *Gerontologist* 23 (1983): 136–143.

16. Kingson, *Ties That Bind,* p. 1.

17. Binstock, "The Aged as Scapegoat," p. 136.

18. Leo W. Simmons, *The Role of the Aged in Primitive Society* (New Haven: Yale University Press, 1945), pp. 42, 82.

19. Karl Barth, *Church Dogmatics,* vol. 3, 4, trans. A. T. Mackay (Edinburgh: T. & T. Clark, 1961), p. 243.

20. M. A. Drickamer and M. S. Lachs, "Should Patients with Alzheimer's Disease Be Told Their Diagnosis?" *New England Journal of Medicine* 326 (1992): 947–951.

21. Joseph M. Foley, "The Experience of Being Demented," in Robert H. Binstock, Stephen G. Post, and Peter J. Whitehouse, eds., *Dementia and Aging: Ethics, Values, and Policy Choices* (Baltimore: Johns Hopkins University Press, 1992), pp. 31–43.

22. F. J. Ingelfinger, "Arrogance," *New England Journal of Medicine* 303 (1980): 1507–1511.

23. Harry R. Moody, *Ethics in an Aging Society* (Baltimore: Johns Hopkins University Press, 1992).

24. Edmund D. Pellegrino and David C. Thomasma, *For the Patient's Good: The Restoration of Beneficence in Health Care* (New York: Oxford University Press, 1988).

25. N. Rango, "The Nursing Home Resident with Dementia: Clinical Care, Ethics, and Policy Considerations," *Annals of Internal Medicine* 102 (1985): 835–841.

26. L. Volicer, "Need for Hospice Approach to Treatment of Patients with Advanced Progressive Dementia," *Journal of the American Geriatrics Association* 34 (1986): 655–658.

27. E. Alemayehu, D. W. Molloy, G. H. Guyatt, "Variability in Physicians' Decisions on Caring for Chronically Ill Elderly Patients: An International Study," *Canadian Medical Association Journal* 144 (1991): 1133–1138.

28. Dan W. Brock, "Justice and the Severely Demented Elderly," *Journal of Medicine and Philosophy* 13, no. 1 (1988): 73.

29. Daniel Callahan, *Setting Limits: Medical Goals in an Aging Society* (New York: Simon and Schuster, 1987), p. 183.

30. R. D. Truog, A. S. Brett, and J. Frader, "The Problem with Futility," *New England Journal of Medicine* 326 (1992): 1560–1564.

31. T. Tomlinson and H. Brody, "Futility and the Ethics of Resuscitation" *Journal of the American Medical Association* 264 (1990): 1277.

32. R. E. Cranford, "Helga Wanglie's Ventilator," *Hastings Center Report* 21, no. 4 (1991): 23–24.

33. Bruce Jennings, "Grassroots Bioethics Revisited: Health Care Priorities and Community Values," *Hastings Center Report* 20, no. 5 (1990): 16.

34. U.S. House of Representatives, Select Committee on Aging, "Paying the Price for Catastrophic Illness: From Accidents to Alzheimer's" (Washington, D.C.: U.S. Government Printing Office, 1987).

35. C. Michelson, M. Mulvihill, M. Hsu, and E. Olson, "Eliciting Medical Care Preferences from Nursing Home Residents," *Gerontologist* 31 (1991): 358–363.

36. Robert Weir, *Selective Nontreatment of Handicapped Newborns* (New York: Oxford University Press, 1984).

37. Robert Katzman, "The Prevalence and Malignancy of Alzheimer Disease," *Archives of Neurology* 33 (1976): 218.

38. Leon Kass, *Toward a More Natural Science: Biology and Human Affairs* (New York: Free Press, 1985).

39. F. Protzman, "Killing of 49 Elderly Patients by Nurse Aids Stuns Austria," *New York Times,* 18 April 1989, p. 1A.

40. John Arras, "The Severely Demented, Minimally Functional Patient: An Ethical Analysis," *Journal of the American Geriatrics Society* 36 (1988): 938–944.

41. Stephen G. Post, "Severely Demented Elderly People: A Case against Senicide," *Journal of the American Geriatrics Society* 38 (1990): 715–718.

42. J. Cohen-Mansfield, J. A. Droge, and N. Billig, "Factors Influencing Hospital Patients' Preferences in the Utilization of Life-sustaining Treatments," *Gerontologist* 32 (1992): 89–95.

43. Robert Applebaum and Paul Phillips, "Assuring the Quality of In-Home Care: The 'Other' Challenge for Long-Term Care," *Gerontologist* 30 (1990): 448.

44. Elaine M. Brody, *Women in the Middle: Their Parent-Care Years* (New York: Springer Publishing, 1990), p. 13.

45. Ibid., pp. 35, 42.

46. Helen Featherstone, *A Difference in the Family* (New York: Basic Books, 1980), pp. 19, 35.

47. Rosalyn Darling, *Families against Society* (Beverley Hills: Sage Library of Social Research, 1979).

48. Brody, *Women in the Middle,* p. 260.

8

The Legacy of Racial Hygiene: Death and Data

Even ardent moral relativists acknowledge that the murderous actions of Nazi doctors during the Holocaust should be universally condemned. What should be the fate of scientific data retrieved from the moral abyss of cruelty and torture, assuming that some such data are empirically valid? Should Nazi data, or any other data gained from atrocity, be left untouched by science? Or can atrocity be, in some sense, redeemed and transcended by salvaging some human benefit from its ashes? Are the victims of atrocity best commemorated by the use of data, or by the categorical rejection of all use?

Methodologically, I examine these questions with an emphasis on the voice of those who are victims of experimental atrocity. My point of departure is Judith N. Shklar's *The Faces of Injustice*. Shklar deeply analyzes the sense of injustice and the desire for revenge on the part of victims. She reaches this conclusion: "Whatever decisions we do make will, however, be unjust unless we take the victim's view into full account and give her voice its full weight."[1] Shklar suggests that unless we hear the victim's voice we remain indifferent to injustice and allow it to continue.

We all know of remarkable harms in human medical experimentation historically. In our own time harms still occasionally occur in the United States and elsewhere, despite the various preventive guidelines and review boards. Unethical human experimentation will continue to emerge until medical scientists deeply hear and respond to the voice of victims, even those whose righteous indignation and resentment are expressed in an

emotional and vengeful manner. Those who have heard the powerful testimony of the survivors of Nazi experiments or of other experimental
atrocities are better for the experience and much less likely to act harm-
fully.

Extrapolating from Shklar's concerns that more philosophical attention is due victims and the notion of injustice, I do not think that the
voice of the victims has been adequately appreciated or interpreted in ethical discussion. For example, a recent collection of writings on research
ethics edited by George J. Annas and Michael A. Grodin, while otherwise
excellent, includes remarkably little of the voice of victims. The editors do
include a testimony from Eva Mozes-Kor, a surviving victim of Nazi medical experimentation who is the president of an international organization,
Children of Auschwitz Nazi Deadly Lab Experiments Survivors (CAN-
DLES). Mozes-Kor was, in her words, "a human guinea pig in the
Birkenau laboratory of Dr. Josef Mengele." In 1944 at age nine she and
her twin sister were swept from their native Transylvanian village into a
world of Mengele's medicalized torture. Among other horrid deeds, Mengele "would inject one twin with the germ. Then, if and when the twin
died, he would kill the other in order to compare the organs at autopsy."
Mozes-Kor almost died after a series of germ injections, but she survived
with her sister for liberation. She provides this pointed description of
atrocity, among others: "A set of Gypsy twins was brought back from
Mengele's lab after they were sewn back to back. Mengele had attempted
to create a Siamese twin by connecting blood vessels and organs. The
twins screamed day and night until gangrene set in, and after three days
they died."[2] Mozes-Kor concludes with an appeal to medical researchers
to respect the dignity of human life and freedom at all costs even when
this delays so-called scientific progress.

The editors should have done more with the voices of victims. Readers might enter into the book more easily through testimonies from survivors highlighted at the very outset, for only they can present the faces of
injustice that elicit immediate compassion, if we accept Shklar's thesis. A
scant six pages of one victim's testimony tucked away after the historians
have waxed eloquent seems inadequate. The call of survivor testimonies
must be the fit beginning of this journey into the abyss, for what else
could be nearly as appropriate?

In general I will oppose usage of Nazi data. I focus on both the importance of deterring future victimization and on sensitivity to the voice of victims themselves, although not all victims are in agreement. Before proceeding, however, I offer opening contextual comments concerning moral disagreement and the symbolic significance of the Nazi data.

Ethics is, as Aristotle claimed, an "inexact science." In most serious moral debates, arguments on both sides are often cogent. Particularly when debates become acrimonious, as the one over Nazi data has become, it must be stressed that differing perspectives are genuine and merit respect.

Within the Jewish community itself, opinion on Nazi data usage is divided. Mark Weitzman of the Simon Wiesenthal Center writes, "As the primary victims of Nazism, Jews have a particular stake in questioning the morality of any profit gained from that system." Weitzman points out that some Jewish thinkers believe using Nazi data makes current researchers "accessories to the crime," relativizes the sense of absolute evil associated with nazism, and could "encourage further inhumane experiments."[3] But Weitzman's own view is that Jewish Law (*Halakhah*) emphasizes the "priority of the ethical," and particularly of the principle that each individual human life is sacred and worthy of preservation. Therefore, if the Nazi data can save a life, it must be used, although the victims should be remembered and the atrocities condemned.[4] Weitzman's position is grounded in Deuteronomy 30:19, "Therefore, choose life," which he thinks should override the deep emotional repugnance that is felt about using anything associated with the Nazis. "I must acknowledge, however, the clear tension between my emotional response and my intellectual position," he notes.[5] I highlight Weitzman's perspective as an example of respectful disagreement on an issue that permits no obvious consensus.

As for Nazi data, what makes them unique, if anything? Many aspects of civilization and progress are built on past knowledge that is morally ambiguous in its origins, if not absolutely condemnable. Can we learn from the architecture of the Egyptians, even though the pyramids were built by millions of slaves who died in the process? Can we benefit from research with fetal tissue taken from elective abortuses, even though we might condemn such abortions, and would Weitzman's perspective apply here by analogy? Human experience lies between the realities of the moral abyss and the ideal of goodness, and in this dialectic much knowledge is tainted. Human achievements occur within the relativities of history, dialectically located between the "impossible possibility" of perfect goodness and the abyss around which we attempt to build fences.[6] The Nazi atrocities are one case among others in which our fence building wholly failed.

No traditions, whether religious or secular, humanistic or scientific, transcend degrees of moral ambiguity. Much moral casuistry involves balancing the "hermeneutics of suspicion" with the "hermeneutics of retrieval."[7] In the process of condemning the moral abyss, how open should we be to the recovery of that which remains useful? In the reality of history, the moral question is rarely, if ever, one of avoiding all taint but rather one of avoiding degrees of taint. We constantly confront the difficult, tragic, and ambiguous aspects of the human condition.

In this sense, the Holocaust and the debate over Nazi data are not *categorically* unique. Yet it remains a fact of modern culture that the Holocaust has taken on a *symbolic* uniqueness as that point where evil converged. As philosophers such as Ernst Cassirer pointed out, the human creation of symbols is a courageous endeavor to deal with problems of meaning and value.[8] The question arises as to whether such a symbol as the Holocaust should be left untouched in order to mark more robustly a boundary between what cultural anthropologists term the domains of the sacred and of the profane. This symbolic boundary is not dealt with in the canons of moral philosophy, but it appears to be important to the way cultures define themselves and develop a sense of integrity, meaning, and well-being.

HUMAN EXPERIMENTATION AND HISTORY

At a recent conference, a survivor of Dr. Josef Mengele's notorious twin experiments argued against data usage because "it is so easy for scientists to step over the edge and make science a God."[9] The survivor warned against the worship of precision, accuracy, and "almighty datum." To use Nazi data, I will contend, is to fail to deter future scientists from further unethical research. This argument of deterrence is mentioned by the editor of the *New England Journal of Medicine,* Marcia Angell, as the first reason why the journal does not publish unethical research.[10]

Judging from history, it is easy for researchers to "step over the edge." With respect to human experimentation, the practices of the Nazi doctors were rather consistent with Western medicine. Atrocity in human experimentation neither began nor ended with Nazi medicine. In 1865 Claude Bernard detailed this history in his classic *An Introduction to the Study of Experimental Medicine,* pointing out that from Galen to Celsus, vivisection inflicted on criminals for the benefit of innocent multitudes was thought appropriate. Bernard provided a host of examples in which physicians experimented with poisons and antidotes on those no longer considered innocent of wrongdoing. He pointed out that "the Grand Duke of Tuscany had a criminal given over to the professor of anatomy, Fallopius, at Pisa, with permission to kill or dissect him at pleasure." In the first known ethical argument against such practices, Bernard constructed this moral rule: "The principle of medical and surgical morality, therefore, consists in never performing on man an experiment that might by harmful to him to any extent, even though the result might be highly advantageous to science, i.e., to the health of others. But performing experiments and operations exclusively from the point of view of the patient's own advantage does not prevent their turning out profitably to science."[11] Bernard insisted that the ground of ethics lies in not "doing ill to one's neighbor," and that this prohibition should hold even though scientific progress might be blocked as a result. The Nuremberg Code followed Bernard in granting nonmaleficence clear lexical priority over even the most well-intentioned efforts to bring about medical and human betterment: "5. No experiment should be conducted where there is an *a priori* reason to believe that death or disabling injury will occur; except, perhaps, in those experiments where the experimental physicians also serve as subjects."[12]

Why has medicine had such difficulty abiding by the fundamental ethical principle "Do no harm" in the context of human experimentation? Perhaps it is because the goal of medical progress is so compelling. Abiding by nonmaleficence requires that some scientific knowledge simply may never be had, at least not in a moral world. In an ethical society, progress attained through harmful means is off-limits, so progress must occur more gradually, if at all in some cases. For researchers, it is especially difficult to come to terms with the notion that medical progress can simultaneously be moral regress.

To a large extent, our culture is utilitarian, and utilitarian empirical scientific reasoning is remarkably powerful. Nevertheless, such reasoning must be restrained, since it so easily allows the ends to justify the means. As Angell concludes, "And finally, refusal to publish unethical work serves notice to society at large that even scientists do not consider science the primary measure of a civilization. Knowledge, although important, may be less important to a decent society than the way it is obtained."[13] Presumably, no researcher will "step over the edge" knowing that there is absolutely nothing to be gained by it for professional or scientific advancement.

It is the widespread concern that medicine has not yet fully and categorically resolved the tension between increasing knowledge and the rejection of harmful means that makes the Nazi data issue so heated. This concern is heightened by recent historical studies of medicine under the Nazis.

RECENT HISTORICAL ASSESSMENT: THE NAZIS AND BEYOND

As stated earlier, recent historical research indicates that the Nazi doctors were not drawn into the abyss against their will. They were continuing a tradition in Western medicine that permitted physicians to inflict harm on social "wrongdoers," a category of persons that could include anyone deviating from social norms, including the religious nonconformist. Had not physicians been present to observe and regulate the torture of the Marranos (Jews whose conversion to Catholicism was allegedly less than genuine), who were the special concern of the Spanish Inquisition?[14]

As Sheila Faith Weiss has recently shown in her study of Wilhelm Schallmayer, M.D., cofounder of the German eugenics movement, racial hygiene theory was the child of social Darwinism. While Schallmayer opposed the racist interpretation of eugenics, he nevertheless fathered the technocratic logic that would actively dispense with all "degenerate" persons, those "unworthy" of life.[15] When he died in 1919, Schallmayer had bequeathed to Germany two categories of human beings, the "valuable" and the "valueless," as well as the assumption that the latter should ultimately be controlled and eliminated. This remains relevant to all discussions of mercy killing.

In another recent work, Robert N. Proctor focuses "not primarily on how the Nazis *corrupted* or *abused* science, but rather on how scientists themselves participated in the construction of Nazi racial policy." According to Proctor, racial hygiene theory was deeply embedded in German biomedical science long before 1933, and German biomedical scientists played an "active, even leading role in the initiation, administration, and execution of Nazi racial programs."[16] Remarkably, Proctor writes as follows:

> The Nazi Physicians' League was an immediate success. By the beginning of 1933 (that is, *before* the rise of Hitler to power), 2,786 doctors had joined the league. Doctors in fact joined the Nazi party earlier and in greater numbers than did any other professional group. The 2,800 doctors joining the league before Hitler's rise to power represented 6 percent of the entire medical profession (whereas only 2.3 percent of all engineers and less than half of one percent of all judges had joined).[17]

As early as the turn of the century, doctors began to develop the discipline of racial hygienics; in the Nazi party they found sympathetic listeners and therefore joined early in higher numbers proportionately than the general population. The doctors were not unwitting victims but, rather, active and responsible agents committed to hygienic theories that legitimized Nazi racial ideology. The historian Michael H. Kater, in a foundational study, shows that while some doctors resisted the Nazi regime's perversion of the healing art, German physicians devoted themselves to Nazi ideology sooner and in much higher numbers than any other professionals, and did more for the regime than their peers.[18]

English and American doctors collaborated with German in making racial hygienics scientifically acceptable. This is especially emphasized in Robert Jay Lifton's study of the Nazi doctors, which points out the extent to which German and American physicians collaborated and provided one another with prestigious awards. Lifton notes that Fritz Lenz, a German physician-geneticist, berated his countrymen in 1923 for "their backwardness in the domain of sterilization as compared with the United States."[19] He complained that Germany had nothing like the American laws prohibiting marriage for people with epilepsy or mental retardation.

American scientists were indeed at the center of the developing field of eugenics. By 1920, twenty-five states required "compulsory sterilization of the criminally insane and other people considered genetically inferior."[20] Interracial marriages were also prohibited. That American physicians were deeply involved in nontherapeutic research resulting in subject death is clear from the Tuskegee Syphilis Study that began in the 1920s. A special panel determined that the Tuskegee study was "not an isolated event in terms of the generally accepted conditions and practices that prevailed in the 1930's."[21] Black men were left untreated after 1953 even though physicians knew that penicillin therapy was effective. As Jay Katz, M.D., has underscored, these experiments continued long after the Nuremberg Code had been widely disseminated to the medical community, and they were not reviewed until public pressure mounted in the late 1960s. The October 1972 issue of the *Southern Medical Journal* exonerated the study and criticized those who brought it to public attention. Katz concludes with this query: "When will we take seriously our responsibilities particularly to the disadvantaged in our midst who so consistently throughout history have been the first to be selected for human research?"[22] So there is wisdom in Reinhold Niebuhr's warning of 1949 that the United States had better avoid vindictiveness and pride in dealing with the "war criminals."[23]

It is significant that although twenty-three German physicians were tried at Nuremberg for crimes against humanity, and seven of them were condemned to death, no similar fate awaited Japanese researchers who carried out equally barbarous experiments in Manchuria between 1930 and 1945.[24] Japan, which was developing sophisticated germ warfare techniques, conducted experiments on prisoners of war to measure physical response to infections. Installations existed near Changchun and Nanjing. Experiments were conducted on the response to "anthrax, botulism, brucellosis, cholera, dysentery, hemorrhagic fever, plague, smallpox, syphilis, tick encephalitis, tsutsugamushi, tularemia, typhoid, and typhus. Other experiments included prolonged exposure to x-rays, freezing body parts to try various methods of thawing, pumping the body full of horse blood, and vivisection."[25] American officials did not prosecute because the Japanese investigators agreed to cooperate with their captors: "A similar fate [to that of the Nazi doctors at Nuremberg] did not await Japanese researchers. . . . Indeed, the existence of these abuses was not even generally known for more than thirty-five years because, in exchange for not being publicly tried and punished, the Japanese investigators agreed to cooperate with their American captors and share information they had gathered about biological warfare through their experiments with Chinese captives."[26] The Japanese physicians were responsible for the deaths of tens of thousands, and their methods were as pernicious as those of the Nazis. America put the data to use in its own biological warfare research.[27]

Along with numerous other nations, the United States fell short of innocence. American medicine was, however, much less guilty than Germany and Japan, and this is meaningful given that all moral achievements of history have been relative rather than absolute. With Niebuhr, we must acknowledge "the equality of sin and the inequality of guilt."[28] Many, certainly not all, physicians of various nations sinned, though some less than others within the relativities of history. They were victims of the will to power that corrupts the will to knowledge, and they hid baser motives in the garb of medical progress. None who sinned was prepared to make that progress subservient to ethical imperatives. "Murderous science" was only more rampant in Germany.[29] It is partly because of a human tendency to condemn others as a way of avoiding self-indictment that the argument of deterrence is so universally relevant.

NAZI DATA AND THE ARGUMENT FROM DETERRENCE

Readers will already be familiar with the atrocious dossier of Nazi experiments ranging from surgical mutilation to phosgene gas exposure. The data were recorded in German wartime medical journals, and some have been cited extensively in the scientific literature since then, particularly in hypothermia studies. Robert L. Berger denounces the usage of these data, claiming that the Dachau hypothermia study "has all the ingredients of a scientific fraud."[30] Indeed, an obvious argument against the usage of data is that they have no scientific validity, and Berger makes a case for this assertion. But even so, the moral question remains: what should be done with unethically obtained data when they are at least in part scientifically valid?

It is remarkable that at Nuremberg the ethical argument of deterrence was not clearly stated. That useful data ought not to be used was never fully considered. The prosecutor, General Telford Taylor, included this statement in his introduction to the case against the German doctors in December of 1946: "Here we leave behind all semblance, however fictitious, of science and research."[31] But this assertion is an expression of moral revulsion, rather than of scientific fact, for Taylor later adds, "These experiments revealed nothing which civilized medicine can use." Taylor maintained that a "civilized medicine" would never stoop so low as to use the Nazi data, but his assertion is undeveloped, as though no one would question it. The absence of any full discussion of data usage had serious ramifications, for researchers were never forced to ask the question of whether to ignore useful data, and they consequently went right ahead and used it. This oversight at Nuremberg, and its troubling repercussions, remain with us "like some morning echo of last night's nightmare."[32]

As early as 1946, the *Journal of the American Medical Association* published a research article entitled "Survival of Hypothermia by Men Immersed in the Ocean," which cites data from the Dachau concentration camp that had been reported in 1945 by Leo Alexander, M.D.[33] The author, G. W. Molnar, devotes eight lengthy paragraphs to a matter-of-fact description of the fatal hypothermia experiments without the slightest pause for moral condemnation. While apologists might say that any sane author or reader would eschew Nazi experimental methods, and that a specific condemnation in the article would therefore be uncalled for, this apology fails. It fails because biomedical research has a tainted history with regard to human experimentation, so a clear condemnation would be reassuring. The article reads like a physics experiment in which human beings are reduced to the status of "thinghood."[34] The reader inevitably wonders if the researcher has lost sight of moral values and human dignity in the pursuit of knowledge. As for the scientific value of the hypothermia data, Molnar states that "these data are considered as objective and valid."[35]

Of the more than forty-five research articles written since 1945 that use Nazi data, most have dealt with hypothermia. If not focused on "cooling curves" measuring fatality rates according to exposure times and temperatures, the articles argue for "rapid external rewarming" as the most effective therapy for accidentally cooled patients.[36] The question remains as to whether it should continue to be cited in the scientific literature. Present-day physiologists still use the figures for cooling, claiming that there does not have to be a correlation between the validity of data and the ethics of the researchers. Useful facts are useful facts, period. Moreover, it is said that only through using the data will the victims not have died in vain.[37]

Robert S. Pozos, a physiologist and former director of the hypothermia laboratory at the University of Minnesota, has been at the center of the controversy over the data's use. He has revised his earlier position favoring use of the Nazi data. He now argues that the data should *not* be referenced any longer in the scientific literature because it sends a message to future researchers that the ends justify the means. This is essentially the argument of deterrence. But only *after* talking with the victims of Nazi medical atrocities did Pozos conclude that the degree of dehumanization and indignation was so great as to outweigh scientific benefit.[38]

Pozos's perspective is similar to that of Henry K. Beecher, who in a now classic article entitled "Ethics and Clinical Research" concludes that data obtained unethically "should not be published." Failure to obtain publication, contends Beecher, would certainly "discourage unethical experimentation," for "how many would carry out such experiments if they *knew* its results would never be published?" Beecher does state that "there is room for debate" as to whether the data should be published with "stern editorial comment" or not published at all. But on balance, he concludes that medical science would suffer a "far-reaching moral loss" if the data were published even with editorial comment. He cites by analogy the legal norm that evidence obtained unconstitutionally cannot be used in any judicial decision.[39]

In contrast to Beecher, Robert J. Levine makes an articulate case for the publication of unethically obtained data. He contends that scientific journals should publish empirically valid but unethically obtained data "along with an editorial in which the ethical questions are raised." The author can be invited to prepare a rebuttal to be published simultaneously. Useful data would thus be saved for science, and unethical researchers would be deeply embarrassed. Levine describes meetings of a committee from the Council of Biology Editors in which a policy of publication or rejection according to the discretion of the individual editor was endorsed. Levine notes that a majority of editors believe it "unethical for an editor to publish unethical research."[40]

The pressure on medical researchers to produce is tremendous, and young researchers who obtain positions find competition for tenure and grants more severe than ever. It is imperative for all researchers to know from the outset of their careers that unethically obtained data will not be of any benefit to them, nor to science.

The hypothermia data that have already been published cannot be "un-learned" or expunged from the journals and texts in which they have already been referenced. Still, current editors could issue a statement apologizing for these publications in their journals and stating clearly that in the future no unethically obtained research data will see the light of print.

One possibility for further deterrence against unethical research has been described by William E. Seidelman. "It has recently been revealed," he writes, "that the remains of victims of Nazi state terror and medical murder have been continuously preserved for anatomical study by some German universities." The institutions involved include the universities of Tübingen, Heidelberg, and Cologne, and the Max Planck Institute of Brain Research. Medical student inquiries are responsible for bringing this fact to public attention. Seidelman calls for burial of the anatomical parts of Nazi victims, an occasion for the "medical community worldwide to confront this legacy and the profession's ongoing potential for evil."[41] It is only now, four decades past Nuremberg, argues Seidelman, that medical science has begun to consider "the ethical implications of using research derived from victimized subjects." Seidelman adds that all medical students and professors in both East and West Germany should attend the burial, and that every medical school in the world should observe the day annually in an appropriate manner.[42] Such an annual ritual would help deter unethical research, but it is highly unlikely that it will ever take place. After all, Hartmut Hanauske-Abel was barred from medical practice by the German Chamber of Physicians for writing "From Nazi Holocaust to Nuclear Holocaust: A Lesson to Learn?" in the English journal *Lancet.*[43]

Thus far I have made a case against the use of data on the basis of the continuing importance of deterring future unethical research, since science is always tempted to "step over the edge" and victimize anew. The history of the accumulation of knowledge, the active participation of doctors in the Nazi phenomenon, and the readiness of American medicine to use tainted data all underscore one essential point: the walls around the moral abyss break down. The more deterrence the better, and toward this end, sensitivity to the plight of those who have been victimized in the past brings one closer to the faces of injustice.

THE PRIORITY OF THE VOICE OF THE VICTIM

Scientific progress must be subservient to those foundational moral prohibitions against harm and deception without which no society can be maintained. In addition to prohibiting the publication of unethically obtained data, deterrence can be furthered by giving greater primacy to the voice of victims. It is here that this essay makes a contribution to the literature.

To be sure, victims of atrocity may themselves disagree about the fate of data. Albert Haas, a physician and survivor of Dachau, endorses usage: "Should the results appear valid, and the decision to use them as the basis for new research be made, the scientist must take every possible opportunity to make clear where and how the original data was collected."[44] There are quite different perspectives and attitudes among the victims, and presumably among their descendants.

But regardless of some difference of opinion, many victims of injustice and cruelty, whatever their religion, race, or nationality, feel categorically that unethical data should be entirely banned from science. This voice can be dismissed as overly sensitive by those who are socially secure and so devoted to "progress" that hearing the cries of victims becomes impossible. The voices of those who have been victimized by medical science have much to contribute to science and to moral civilization.

To my knowledge, no literature on the ethics of experimentation has yet accounted for the voice of victims, of those whose bodies and souls have been ruthlessly tortured. Yet it is the victims—and possibly their descendants—who should have a say in the fate of data cruelly extracted from them. This is because many victims are harmed yet again by data usage.

Mozes-Kor states the following:

> In Auschwitz we were treated like a commodity: the hair was used for mattresses; the fat was used for soap; the skin for lampshades; the gold collected from the teeth of the dead went into the Nazi treasury, and many of us were used as guinea pigs. Today some doctors want to use the only thing left by these victims. They are like vultures waiting for the corpses to cool so they could devour every consumable part. To use the Nazi data is obscene and sick. One can always rationalize that it would save human lives, the question should be asked at what cost?[45]

Kor adds, "In the case of Mengele Twins, copy of the data should be given to those twins who are still alive," and data of victims who are dead should be "shredded and placed in a transparent monument, as evidence that they exist, but cannot be used." This would be a lesson to the world that "human dignity and human life are more important than any advance in science or medicine."[46] One is reminded of a statement by a black South African physician in regard to data unethically obtained from black prisoners: "I, categorically, yes categorically, as a physician and as a human being, will have absolutely nothing to do with it."[47]

The violation of human dignity is, alas, common. It is an unhappy fact that we all, rather constantly, benefit directly or indirectly from the suffering of others. Victims of atrocity should be heard because they remind the world of its nearness to the abyss. Hearing their voices, we often respond with a categorical imperative, like the South African mentioned above. The Holocaust victims force us to feel some of the actual anguish that torments them, and to acknowledge that data really are in that peculiar category of the profane and untouchable.

Hearing victims shocks one into asking whether the Nazi data even belong to science, any more than slaveholders own or possess goods created through the forced labor of slaves. It is reasonable to think that African Americans abused in American medical studies on syphilis conducted at Tuskegee should have the say as to whether that data should be destroyed or used. Many African Americans, I surmise, would find any use of such data repulsive, for use can be viewed as a continuation of past injustice. Their wishes should be respected, for to override their perspective would be to violate consent doubly—that is, not only in the experimental process itself but in its aftermath. Doubtless those who are committed to utilitarian medical progress will find the voice of the oppressed to be "oversensitive," but this wholly predictable response is characteristic of all those who have not themselves felt the sting of oppression.

It is precisely in the aftermath of unethical experimentation that some opportunity to restore respect and rights to the victims presents itself. To use the data without the consent of those who tragically call it their own is to violate the violated. Let the following maxim be proposed: those who have been experimented on without consent have the ultimate right and authority to pass final judgment on the fate of data. Through tragedy, the victims hold a certain unchallengeable right to control the data. Who, in good conscience, would want seriously to challenge those who have suffered so much at the hands of scientific research? Here the victims of Dachau are no more special or unique than any other victims of the unrestrained will to knowledge.

American medicine could establish a special committee that would allow victims' voices to be heard and published widely, a Committee for the Victims of Experimental Atrocity. It could be made up of leaders in American medicine, along with representative victims, including African Americans, American Indians, Jews, the disabled, the elderly, and any other relevant groups. This committee would disseminate to physicians the testimonies and perspectives of victims and encourage serious consideration of these voices. There is good reason to publish the testimonies of victims in medical journals so that researchers can relate to the anguish of victimization and review even more thoroughly their own research ethics.

Perhaps such a committee of victims would consider the use of unethically obtained data if the benefit to humanity were on a *very* high order of magnitude, for instance, a cure for AIDS or cancer. With such a committee, victimized groups would feel a part of the process of consent and decision, so that any possible rare exception to the argument from deterrence would not then constitute or be perceived by them as further abuse.

A POSTLUDE

When we look back at medical experimentation throughout the course of history, when we reflect on centuries of torture, when we consider the actions of physicians in this century in particular, the only reasonable response is "never again." In order to ensure a better future for society and for the medical profession, it is necessary to hold, as an absolute maxim, that no unethically obtained data shall see the light of publication. Only this message raises moral standards within medicine so high that no physicians will again fall so low. After all, as Richard Rubenstein and John Roth underscore, the Holocaust "was a new kind of *civilized,* legalized" destructiveness, and presumably what happened once can happen again.[48]

Any possible exceptions to this maxim should be made in collaboration with representative victims of scientific atrocities. Such representatives, of whatever race or nationality, understand the emotional scars that victims carry. They might rarely, if ever, grapple with a case in which the magnitude of possible human benefit is so remarkably high that the wall of deterrence would be briefly lifted. They would be always suspicious of the characteristic tendency of researchers to exaggerate the importance of their work. By partial analogy, if fetal tissue transplant really does provide a reliable cure for some neurodegenerative diseases, then some defense of it is possible as long as guidelines prevent payment for abortion and preclude women from designating a recipient.

Finally, a concluding rejoinder. It has been said to me that the prohibition suggested here is too strict, for after all, even the Jewish physicians were themselves involved in experimentation in the Warsaw ghetto. The Warsaw ghetto period lasted approximately two years. The Nazis had sealed off several hundred thousand Jews from the outside world, determined to starve them to death. Partly because some food was successfully smuggled into the ghetto, the Nazis resorted to massive deportation and concentration camps in February of 1942. It is true that Jewish physicians in the five-month period prior to the deportation engaged in research on "hunger disease." As Myron Winick, M.D., writes in his preface to a remarkable book originally published in Polish in 1946 and entitled *Hunger Disease: Studies by the Jewish Physicians in the Warsaw Ghetto,* "The book you are about to read is one that is, and that we can only hope will remain, unique in the annals of medicine. It is the report of a scientific study by physicians condemned to die of the same disease they were studying—hunger and subsequent starvation."[49] The major figure in organizing the study was Israel Milejkowski, the Jewish physician responsible for public health in the ghetto. His motivation was partly scientific, although chiefly moral: "He felt that it was necessary for the world to know the extent and crippling consequences of the starvation being imposed."[50] Of the twenty-eight physicians who participated, their fates were uniformly tragic. Emil Apfelbaum alone survived to recover the buried manuscript and prepare it for publication just before his death in 1946. Of the manuscript content, Winick concludes thus: "The clinical observations in both children and adults constitute probably the best clinical description of the effects of severe semistarvation published in the medical literature to that date and perhaps even to the present."[51] There were 43,000 deaths from starvation.

It must be underscored that these data were obtained *ethically.* As Winick rightly insists, "The investigators were above all physicians, dedicated to the art of healing."[52] They tried desperately to keep people alive, even resorting to blood transfusions. These physicians simply made observations and measurements consistent with beneficent medical practice. Despite the Nazi atrocities, these physicians were able to carry on their work as a tribute to medicine at its best. As Milejkowski wrote in his introduction, "A last few words to honor you, the Jewish doctors. What can I tell you, my beloved colleagues and companions in misery. You are a part of all of us. Slavery, hunger, deportation, those death figures in our ghetto were also your legacy. And you by your work could give the henchman the answer, 'Non omnis moriar,' 'I shall not wholly die.'"[53]

NOTES

1. Judith N. Shklar, *The Faces of Injustice* (New Haven: Yale University Press, 1990), p. 126.

2. Eva Mozes-Kor, "The Mengele Twins and Human Experimentation: A Personal Account," in George J. Annas and Michael A. Grodin, eds., *Nazi Doctors and the Nuremberg Code: Human Rights in Human Experimentation* (New York: Oxford University Press, 1992), pp. 56, 57.

3. Mark Weitzman, "The Ethics of Using Nazi Medical Data: A Jewish Perspective," *Second Opinion: Health, Faith, and Ethics* 14 (July 1990): 30, 31.

4. Ibid., p. 33.

5. Ibid., p. 36.

6. I take this theme of the moral dialectic, and the notion of the moral ideal as paradoxically an "impossible possibility," from the Protestant ethicist Reinhold Niebuhr's many writings.

7. See David Tracy, *The Analogical Imagination* (New York: Crossroad, 1983).

8. Ernst Cassirer, *An Essay on Man* (New Haven: Yale University Press, 1944); see also Paul Ricouer, *The Symbolism of Evil* (Boston: Beacon Press, 1969).

9. Susan Vigorito, from a paper read at the Ninth Annual Holocaust Conference, Kent State University, 20 March 1990.

10. Marcia Angell, "The Nazi Hypothermia Experiments and Unethical Research Today," *New England Journal of Medicine* 322, no. 20 (1990): 1462.

11. Claude Bernard, *An Introduction to the Study of Experimental Medicine*, reprinted in Stanley Joel Reiser, Arthur J. Dyck, and William J. Curran, eds., *Ethics in Medicine: Historical Perspectives and Contemporary Concerns* (Cambridge: MIT Press, 1977), pp. 257–258.

12. "The Nuremberg Code," in Reiser, Dyck, and Curran, *Ethics in Medicine*, p. 273.

13. Angell, "Nazi Hypothermia Experiments," p. 1464.

14. See Cecil Roth, *A History of the Marranos* (New York: Schocken Books, 1974).

15. Sheila Faith Weiss, *Race, Hygiene, and National Efficiency: The Eugenics of Wilhelm Schallmayer* (Berkeley: University of California Press, 1987), p. 150.

16. Robert N. Proctor, *Racial Hygiene: Medicine under the Nazis* (Cambridge: Harvard University Press, 1988), pp. 3, 6.

17. Ibid., p. 65.

18. Michael H. Kater, *Doctors under Hitler* (Chapel Hill: University of North Carolina Press, 1989).

19. Robert Jay Lifton, *The Nazi Doctors: Medical Killing and the Psychology of Genocide* (New York: Basic Books, 1986), p. 23.

20. Ibid., p. 22.

21. *Final Report of the Tuskegee Syphilis Study Ad Hoc Advisory Panel*, in Reiser, Dyck, and Curran, *Ethics in Medicine*, p. 320.

22. Jay Katz, "Reservations about the Panel Report on Charge 1," in Reiser, Dyck, and Curran, *Ethics in Medicine*, p. 321.

23. Reinhold Niebuhr, "What Is Justice?" in D. B. Robertson, ed., *Love and Justice: Selections from the Shorter Writings of Reinhold Niebuhr* (Gloucester, Mass.: Peter Smith, 1976), pp. 229–231.

24. See Alexander M. Capron, "Human Experimentation," in Robert Veatch, ed., *Medical Ethics* (Boston: Jones and Bartlett, 1989), pp. 126–172.

25. Ibid., p. 138.

26. See R. Gomer, J. Powell, and B. Roling, "Japan's Biological Weapons: 1930–1945," *Bulletin of the Atomic Scientist* 37, no. 8 (1981), as cited by Capron, "Human Experimentation," p. 138.

27. Ibid.

28. Reinhold Niebuhr, *The Nature and Destiny of Man*, vol. 1 (New York: Charles Scribner's Sons, 1941), p. 219.

29. See Benno Muller-Hill, *Murderous Science: Elimination by Scientific Selection of Jews, Gypsies, and Others: Germany 1933–35* (New York: Oxford University Press, 1988).

30. Robert L. Berger, "Nazi Science—The Dachau Hypothermia Experiments," *New England Journal of Medicine* 322, no. 20 (17 May 1990): 1435–1440.

31. Telford Taylor, in *Trials of War Criminals before Nuremberg Military Tribunals under Control Council Law No. 10*, vol. 1 (Washington, D.C.: U.S. Government Printing Office, 1956).

32. Reinhold Niebuhr, "What Is Justice?" p. 229.

33. G. W. Molnar, "Survival of Hypothermia by Men Immersed in the Ocean," *Journal of the American Medical Association* 131, no. 13 (27 July 1946): 1046–1050.

34. Hans Jonas, "Philosophical Reflections on Experimenting with Human Subjects," in Reiser, Dyck, and Curran, *Ethics in Medicine*, pp. 304–315.

35. Molnar, "Survival of Hypothermia," p. 1047.

36. See John P. Fernandez, Robert A. O'Rourke, and Gordon A. Ewy, "Rapid Active External Rewarming in Accidental Hypothermia," *Journal of the American Medical Association* 212, no. 1 (6 April 1970): 153–155.

37. See Bernard Dixon, "Citations of Shame," *New Scientist* 105, no. 1445 (28 February 1985): 31.

38. Robert S. Pozos, "Scientific Inquiry and Ethics: The Dachau Data," in Arthur L. Caplan, ed., *When Medicine Went Mad: Bioethics and the Holocaust* (Totowa, N.J.: Humana Press, 1992), pp. 95–108.

39. Henry K. Beecher, "Ethics and Clinical Research," *New England Journal of Medicine*, in Reiser, Dyck, and Curran, *Ethics in Medicine*, pp. 288–293.

40. Robert J. Levine, *Ethics and Regulation of Clinical Research* (New Haven: Yale University Press, 1988), pp. 28, 31.

41. William E. Seidelman, "In Memoriam: Medicine's Confrontation with Evil," *Hastings Center Report* 19, no. 6 (November/December 1989): 5, 6.

42. Ibid., p. 5.

43. Hartmut Hanauske-Abel, "From Nazi Holocaust to Nuclear Holocaust: A Lesson to Learn?" *Lancet* 2 (August 1986): 271-273.

44. Albert Haas, "Ethics Where There Are None," *N.Y.U. Physician* 45, no. 1 (Fall 1988): 67.

45. Eva Mozes-Kor, "Nazi Experiments as Viewed by a Survivor of Mengele's Experiments," in Arthur L Caplan, ed., *When Medicine Went Mad,* p. 7.

46. Ibid.

47. This statement was made at the American Public Health Association National Meeting, Chicago, 24 October 1989, in the panel session "Ethical Issues in the Publication of Nazi Data."

48. Richard L. Rubenstein and John K. Roth, *Approaches to Auschwitz: The Holocaust and Its Legacy* (Atlanta: John Knox Press, 1987), p. 340.

49. Myron Winick, Preface to *Hunger Disease: Studies by the Jewish Physicians in the Warsaw Ghetto,* ed. Myron Winick, trans. Martha Osnos (New York: Wiley, 1979), p. vii.

50. Ibid.

51. Ibid., p. x.

52. Ibid.

53. Israel Milejkowski, "Introduction" to Winick, *Hunger Disease,* p. 5.

9

The Emergence of Species Impartiality: A Medical Critique of Biocentrism

That human beings ought not to inflict pain on sentient animals goes without saying. This proscription underlies the policy statements of the National Institutes of Health regarding humane care and use of laboratory animals.[1] Humane treatment of animals, however, does not require species impartiality, the view that all sentient animal species are of equal moral standing, including human beings. Otherwise, one would have to agree with Paul Taylor that human beings have no greater worth than other species, since any claim to greater worth based on human capacities is judged from the human viewpoint, whereas from the perspective of a tree greater longevity is the value-making capacity, and from the viewpoint of a cheetah, speed. Thus does Taylor arrive at the "principle of species impartiality."[2] Most prominent philosophers of animal rights or liberation in fact do not defend species impartiality; they contend only that animal pain of a certain intensity and duration is as important as human pain of the same intensity and duration and should be avoided with equal consideration.

Yet species impartiality is an emerging and no longer peripheral philosophy, according to which human lives count for no more morally than do nonhuman. Thus Alan Wolfe laments "an emerging anti-humanist cosmology that is profoundly different in its ethical implications from popular environmental views."[3] He is careful not to attribute this cosmology to the animal rights or liberation theorists generally. Willard Gaylin

does include such theorists in his wider critique, arguing that "the reputa-
tion of our species is also under attack, in a way that is half direct and half
indirect, through what has come to be known as the animal rights movement." Animal rights or liberation theorists intend "to protect the beast,"
which Gaylin views favorably, but "in so doing they seriously undermine
the special nature of being human."[4] In fact, Gaylin may overstate the
point, since animal rights and liberation theorists, although opposed to
cruelty and pain, generally acknowledge that the capacities of normal
human beings do count for greater value. Nevertheless, Gaylin's point, as
Wolfe's, merits serious attention.

The basic choice is between (a) a reasonable anthropocentrism, that
is, partiality to human beings that avoids unnecessary or cruel use of animals, and (b) a biocentrism in which all partiality for humans is casti-
gated. A reasonable anthropocentrism maintains that animals, insofar as
they are sentient beings capable of experiencing pain, should receive moral
consideration. Any moral philosophy that denies this is inconsistent and
can be used to justify cruelty. Torture of animals, in experimentation or
any setting, is morally wrong; humane use of animals must be for clearly
beneficial human purposes. It is not obvious that, as one author suggests,
"the current animal-rights movement threatens the future of health science far more than many physicians recognize."[5] The avoidance of pain
and unnecessary sacrifice of animals in research does not entail the cessa-
tion of animal use. Moreover, theorists of animal rights would generally
disagree with an extreme and oft-cited statement from a leader of People
for the Ethical Treatment of Animals: "There is no rational basis for sepa-
rating out the human animal. A rat is a pig is a dog is a boy. They're all
mammals."[6] The not-very-critical activist factions can be distinguished
from the philosophers making the strongest contributions to our understanding of these matters. Peter Singer, for example, while convinced that
pain suffered by sentient animals is as morally significant as that experienced by *Homo sapiens*, quickly adds, "This does not mean that a human
being and a mouse must always be treated equally, or that their lives are of
equal value."[7]

It is biocentrism rather than reasonable anthropocentrism that is of
concern in this chapter. Deep ecology is the chief example of biocentrism.
Some ecofeminism would also qualify.[8] Biocentrism embraces species

impartiality; it rejects even important and painless research on animals; and it suggests that the human pursuit of truth, goodness, and beauty does not set us apart from other species (including plants) in a profound way. I will explain biocentrism in greater detail in the next section.

True, humans should avoid anthropocentric dizziness, because it can result in torture of animals. But the question, How should humans think of themselves? still remains. If the human species is superior to others because of its unique capacities, then species membership is significant, and it is a ground for rejecting biocentric species impartiality. How any entity is valued and treated depends on its nature. If not, then were the choice necessary, one might as well rescue an owl rather than an imperiled neighbor.

BIOCENTRIC SPECIES IMPARTIALISM: THE CURRENT DEBATE

What vexes me is a kind of creeping Jainism, although in modern garb. This ancient religion from India distinguishes only between two kinds of entity, those that possess life (*jiva*) and those that do not (*ajiva*). Coupled with the principle of nonviolence (*ahimsa*), Jainas proscribe even the painless sacrifice of animals for clearly significant human purposes. Their biocosmology disallows any moral distinctions except between the animate and the inanimate.[9]

The modern garb of Jainism is deep ecology, which so values the biosphere that the use of animals for well-founded human purposes is rejected as hubris. Deep ecologists believe that each and every living thing has intrinsic value giving it a right to flourish regardless of usefulness to human beings. They distinguish themselves from shallow ecologists, that is, from practical reformers who still allow that human beings can manipulate other living things in ways that are useful. A prominent philosopher of deep ecology, Arne Naess, argues for "biospherical egalitarianism," the "equal right to live and blossom." J. Baird Callicot defends the similar view, "axiological complementarity."[10] A related position suggests that John Rawls's theory of justice be extended, so that Rawls's "veil of ignorance" conceals the species of those behind it.[11] One animal rights theorist, Michael Fox, argues for human-nonhuman impartiality according to the affinities of sentient animals with humans, including morphological likeness, similarities of origin (ancestral convergence), likeness of experience, and likeness in ability.[12] Continuities between human and nonhuman are exaggerated, discontinuities ignored.

Either implicitly or explicitly, the proponents of species impartiality would understand the fate of a laboratory rat to be as poignant as that of a child's. Medical researchers are not wrong simply because they may do unnecessary or cruel research on animals but because they do research at all. In short, one species, ours, has no right to use other species to solve our health problems.[13] As for medical progress, the response is that we need less of it.[14] On the popular level, this sentiment is echoed in the opposition to cutting down trees containing a chemical that may well cure ovarian cancer, lest the ecological niche of an owl or moth be compromised. Such a view is consistent with James Lovelock's "Gaia hypothesis" in which all living things count equally, from whales to weeds.[15]

A ground swell of species-impartiality sentiment is perhaps an undercurrent among those activists who oppose animal research, even if the major philosophers of animal rights or liberation are separate from it. In response to species impartiality, John Kleinig writes that we should not inflict pain on animals, "but equally, when caring about and interpreting animal behavior, there may be a strong temptation to construct their lives and experience analogously to our own, even though the evidence for doing so is at best problematic." He adds that "we are not dealing with a simple continuity from animal to human experience: some differences in degree make for differences in kind."[16] Common evolutionary origins and morphological similarity independent of *capacity*, he contends, carry no moral weight. The impartialists rightly reject the infliction of pain on animals, but this does not require the abolition of painless killing. "What we should avoid, however, is the easy anthropomorphizing of animals to which the cartoon world of childhood fantasies may incline us," Klienig warns.[17]

Similarly, the philosopher Michael P. T. Leahy argues that human beings wrongly attribute strictly human qualities to nonhuman sentient species. In a broad criticism of animal liberationists, Leahy analyzes anthropomorphism, the depiction of animals as more than they are. He assesses a wide literature describing the fate of laboratory animals, designed "to evoke chilling reminders of men, women, and children huddled in ghastly expectation; dying in pogroms and concentration camps." But, Leahy contends, animals remain unaware of their fate, having neither an understanding of dying nor a self-conscious desire to live. Killing animals for necessary laboratory research "will only seem immoral if (yet again) there is a confused identification with similar programs were they to involve human beings." Killing an animal does harm it, Leahy adds, but so does "cutting down a tree."[18]

THE ARGUMENT FOR PARTIALITY

Species impartialists echo the refrain that human beings must moderate their pretensions and admit that they are a little animal living a precarious existence. This is not new. Four centuries ago, Michel de Montaigne, inspired by Plutarch, made precisely this point in his famous "Apology for Raimond Sebond (Man's Presumption and Littleness)," in which a "miserable and puny creature," the "frailest and most vulnerable of all creatures," human beings, are chastised for mistakenly presuming a central place in the universe.[19] Such views serve to challenge species arrogance and insensitivity to the sufferings of nonhumans and to remind us of our dependence on the ecosystem. But if human beings have superior capacities and assert that they are superior beings, they are not arrogant but veracious. The problem lies only in drawing unwarranted practical inferences from this superiority, for example, in justifying cruelty to nonhumans.

It must be acknowledged that in this world, humans are the only known moral agents, that is, beings to whom we may meaningfully ascribe moral obligations, and therefore are beings of rational reflection. Animals are, as philosophers use the term, "moral patients," that is, with respect to the removal of pain they count morally for their own sake and not simply because of the consequences for humans of treating them cruelly. To treat sentient beings in a manner appropriate to their nature means not to inflict suffering. But animals are not persons in the sense that they are not endowed with the capacity for moral agency. Because we are endowed with free choice and the capacity to reflect on and morally evaluate our free choices (conscience), we hold ourselves and one another accountable for freely chosen actions. Superiority of nature must be action guiding, that is, counted in judging higher degrees of moral considerability. Perhaps apes could be trained to use symbols, but this does not mean that they engage in abstract reasoning or have moral agency. Reaching back into religious mythology, what separates humans from all other beings on earth is the capacity to distinguish between good and evil.

An adequate ethical system must include "respect" for sentient beings as such insofar as they merit moral consideration, or freedom from pain. But human beings as moral agents are entitled to a greater respect. Humans can further be seen to differ from animals in at least five important ways: first, the development of languages in which meanings are understood and communicated; second, the presence of historical consciousness—the awareness of the past and the awareness that we do not simply repeat what we have done in the past; third, the construction of a culture that even in "primitive" and subsistence societies involves the use of materials manipulated in a symbolic fashion; fourth, self-consciousness in the strict sense, that is, awareness of oneself as a self, which makes possible and makes sense of first-person statements; and fifth, the quest for meaning. These five factors, but particularly moral agency, allow a uniquely high evaluation of human beings in relation to other sentient beings, so the painless taking of the life of a member of another species in order to ensure human welfare would be moral.

SPECIES LOYALTY

Yet what about our common moral commitments to human beings whose relevant capacities are below those of some animals, for example, newborns or people with advanced progressive dementia? The moral pull of members of our own species should still exert greater weight on us as agents than the pull of beings outside our species. This claim rests on a notion of species loyalty that extends to human beings categorically, not only to those human beings who possess certain intact capacities.

There must be a defense of those human beings who are not fully intact against those who would reverse common morality. Cognitively marginal human beings may not reason or act as moral agents, may have limited relational capacities and communication skills, and may not seek meaning in life. Patients in the persistent vegetative state or who suffer from advanced dementia do not manifest any obvious superiority of nature over certain nonhuman sentient species, but they are nevertheless members of *our* species. Through providing them with comfort care we solidify a categorical loyalty to one another that should not be compromised. David H. Smith worries that personhood theories of ethics, which focus on developed human capacities such as reasoning, memory, and purposefulness as grounds for moral considerability, can become an "engine of exclusion" of many human beings from moral consideration. Smith, in an account of caring for his mother-in-law as she deteriorated from Alzheimer's disease, emphasizes that loyalty and essential moral sentiments dictate comfort care that theories focusing on intact capacities do not require.[20]

Of course appeals to prereflexive moral intuitions and to common morality are problematic, for they may reflect biases. More argument is needed. In this section, I wish to make a point about the ordering of moral obligations, especially with respect to beneficence. Although justice requires stricter impartiality, obligations of beneficence allow for considerable partiality. One can accept the idea that we should extend our beneficence to humans before nonhumans because of our species loyalty but deny that this loyalty allows us the liberty to inflict cruelty on animals. Although we have an obligation not to do harm to members of nonhuman sentient species, our fellow humans by virtue of their proximity to us have a stronger claim on our beneficence.

Christina Hoff Sommers, in an essay dealing with filial obligations, refers to Mrs. Jellyby, a character in Charles Dickens's *Bleak House,* who "devotes all of her considerable energies to the foreign poor to the complete neglect of her family." She points out that "Before the turn of the century there was no question that a filial relationship defined a natural obligation; philosophers argued about the nature of filial obligation, but not about its reality." Sommers's basic theme is that Enlightenment and post-Enlightenment ethical theory, both deontological and utilitarian, does not easily account for ordered obligations based on kinship. These theories, continues Sommers, "seem better designed for telling us what we should do for everyone impartially than for explaining something like filial obligations."[21]

I believe that species membership is analogous to family membership and is the basis of obligations that take precedence over, but do not negate, obligations to nonmembers. Obligations of beneficence are impartial only in the most abstract way; in real life, our obligations are laid down in a flexible hierarchy and are to be fulfilled proportionately.

Sommers states that in contemporary ethics, moral obligation has been reduced to one level of "equal pull," in which familial relations are no more binding on moral agents than the claims of strangers. She sees this as counterintuitive, like a gravitational field in which gravitational force has been equalized, so the pull of planets more distant from one another is equal to the pull of planets in proximity. Sommers finds this equalization inconsistent with moral experience, where our understanding of our obligations is based on "differential pull," that is, of special obligations to those in proximity.

Michael Walzer has criticized efforts to deny special obligations. He writes that, contrary to the strict impartialist, "the rest of us must settle for something less, which we are likely to think of as something better: we draw the best line that we can between the family and the community and live with the unequal intensities of love."[22] Walzer reminds us that however much saints and hermits choose to ignore the moral importance of ordered obligations based on special relationships and proximity, most of us in practice and everyday life affirm their importance. Certainly between extreme impartiality and extreme partiality is a plausible middle ground.

Our species kinship creates special obligations of justice and beneficence that take precedence over our obligations to members of other species. It is possible that my relations with a human stranger are less affectionate than those with my dog, Spot, but they are more compelling and morally weighty. I may have great affection for Spot, but it remains a moral wrong to save Spot rather than an abandoned baby, were the choice necessary. Common morality and good Samaritan laws would judge me grossly negligent were I to ignore the infant. Our shared species membership constitutes a moral field that rightly demands and should receive priority even over my special feelings for Spot. A human is a human; a dog is a dog. (Were we to reject ordered obligations based on species membership, then we could take much of the $900 billion currently spent each year in this country for human health care and shift it to acute and long-term animal care.)

Sociobiological literature would support the notion of species loyalty. Human affective and social capacities are understood as the outgrowth of millennia of human evolution shaped by natural selection. In this enlarged time framework, "kin selection" or "kin altruism" is deeply ingrained in the human "biogram." "Hard core altruism," as Edward O. Wilson defines it, is directed toward close kin, and "expresses no desire for equal return."[23] There is thus a certain order of beneficence that provides primary familial relations with a high moral priority. Although this does not imply that reasoning and free human beings must place an imprimatur on moral parochialism, it does attach value to the "natural" orderings of life.[24] The sociobiological context indicates how natural selection directs human moral commitments to the human species, although this does not mean that humans should not have concern about the welfare of nonhuman species. Yet the simplest reflection on what any species is indicates that it will have certain crucial inclinations and tendencies that mold an inherent preference for itself.

According to some philosophers, such tendencies have no ethical significance, for values cannot be derived from facts, or, more technically, *ought* cannot be derived from *is* (the "naturalistic fallacy"). Therefore, they argue that no matter how much sociobiology tells us about what we as a species are in terms of evolutionary adaptations, this is ethically irrelevant. This debunks the ethical significance of kin or reciprocal altruism and favors a strictly "rational" utilitarian starting point of disinterested impartiality that sees special obligations and partialities as emotional obstacles to moral progress. But Bernard Williams offers a powerful criticism of the impartialism that strips the self of its embeddedness in biological and communal realities (albeit somewhat flexible ones). In his classic rebuttal of such impartialism, he writes that an ethics that strips the moral agent of special relations and commitments forces a rift between the agent and his or her deepest moral projects.[25] Hence, it is not philosophically outlandish to consider the pull of partiality as morally significant.

I am attempting to develop a positive interpretive framework here for a position that is widely held and that has been articulated concisely by Carl Cohen: "I am a speciesist. Speciesism is not merely plausible; it is essential for right conduct, because those who will not make the morally relevant distinctions among species are almost certain, in consequence, to misapprehend their true obligations. The analogy between speciesism and racism is insidious." Racism, writes Cohen, "has no moral ground whatsoever," since there are no morally relevant differences between the races. Between species of animate life, however—for example, humans and rats—"the morally relevant differences are enormous, and almost universally appreciated."[26] Cohen goes on to list human capacities, such as rationality, that distinguish humans from nonhumans. The term "speciesism" to which Cohen responds is attributed to Singer, whose most recent definition is this: "a prejudice or attitude of bias in favor of the interests of member's of one's own species and against those of members of other species. It should be obvious that the fundamental objections to racism and sexism made by Thomas Jefferson and Sojourner Truth apply equally to speciesism."[27] I too am a speciesist and find the analogies to racism and sexism indefensible.

But I want to go even further than Cohen, to include a moral primacy for human beings even when they lack certain capacities that fulfill various "indicators of personhood." A human being may lack a sense of personal history, self-identity, and meaning; he or she may lack various cognitive and communicative capacities; but I would nevertheless provide comfort care for that vulnerable and incompetent human rather than for a perfectly intact nonhuman were the choice imposed. Our commitment to the family of humanity necessarily rejects species impartiality, and this rejection is appropriate. Moral agents ought to treat moral patients of the same species differently from moral patients of other species. Humans have special obligations to other humans that require no apologies. Only an exceedingly abstract philosophy of the self would suggest otherwise. To save an abandoned baby rather than an adult monkey is morally incumbent on human beings. This does not constitute some new prejudicial "ism" akin to racism or sexism. Our relations to and duties toward other humans define, partially at least and sometimes wholly, our obligations and duties.

Nel Noddings, who also opposes cruelty to animals, develops the theme of "primary obligation" based on human affections and the roots of "ethicality." She writes as follows: "Locating our primary obligation in the domain of human life is a logical outgrowth of the fact that ethicality is defined in the human domain—that the moral attitude would not exist or be recognized without human affection and rational reflection upon or assessment of that affection. It is not 'speciesism' to respond differently to different species if the very form of the response is species specific."[28] She acknowledges that animals should be treated kindly and sensitively, but human commitments to other humans retain priority.

We have swung too far away from theorists such as Thomas Aquinas, Joseph Butler, Adam Ferguson, Adam Smith, and Henry Sidgwick, who believed firmly in "the Order in which Individuals are recommended by Nature to our care and attention."[29] Just as it is reasonable to do more first for those closest to us for whom we are particularly responsible, so also it is reasonable to do good for human beings first, simply as such, and then for members of nonhuman species, when the unfortunate choice is necessary. Affection for animals can create deep emotional bonds, and these bonds are good insofar as they prevent cruelty. But let us be skeptical of any emotional bonds with members of nonhuman species that would result in overturning appropriate preference when human life must be saved. Our obligations toward other humans are categorically most weighty.

It is by natural inclination, deeply reinforced by moral and religious tradition, that human beings have a moral partiality toward their own species. As John Benson argues against Singer, "Partiality for our own species, and within it for much smaller groupings, is, like the universe, something we had better accept. That we care at all about the interests of strangers of our own species or animals of other species results from our extending to them by sympathy something of the concern that we feel spontaneously for those with whom we have closer connections."[30]

FURTHERING THE ETHICAL

Human beings should be valued and treated consistently with their nature and capacities. We humans are higher beings, with a sovereignty that resides above the whole mass of sentient species; privilege belongs to some things more than others. Partiality in this context is not analogous to sexism or racism, for these are rooted in prejudice and false claims of difference, rather than in veracity.

With respect to human beings who are cognitively incapacitated or undeveloped, we as members of the human species have duties of beneficence such that our first, though not our only, obligations are to our

fellow humans. I am aware of R. G. Frey's argument that species membership is not a ground for "a special moral relationship to our fellow
humans," since such membership is not voluntary, and voluntariness is a
feature of special relations. Because "my own choices and decisions have
no effect on species membership," Frey continues, such membership is "at
odds not only with how we typically understand special moral relationships but also with how we typically understand our relationship to our
own morality."[31] Frey's argument is relevant only to friendships, however,
not to the familial relationships that we are born into. Moreover, the various moral theorists cited in my discussion of special obligations would
uniformly disagree with Frey's precondition of voluntariness, since they
see such obligations as given by nature.

People may not use the greater respect due to moral agents and the
necessary species ordering of beneficence as an excuse for harming sentient
beings, which, as such, have a claim not to be gratuitously harmed. Because cruelty toward members of nonhuman species has occurred often in
the course of history, it is in one sense good that species impartialism has
emerged. But species impartialism leaves us with a badly distorted model
of the real world of rights and obligations. Such a position is antihuman,
even if unintentionally so. All eco-wholistic worldviews, which view human beings as a part of the whole with no preeminence within it, ultimately are stumbling blocks for medical progress and the human good.

BABOON LIVERS AND THE HUMAN GOOD

The prospects for successfully transplanting a baboon liver into a human
being have been raised by Dr. Thomas E. Starzl's well-publicized recent
case in which a baboon liver was transplanted into a thirty-five-year-old
man who died seventy-one days later after a stroke. It was thought that
the patient's hepatitis, which would attack any human liver, would be
unable to attack a baboon liver. Starzl's planned future transplants will
clarify this point.[32] I only raise an underlying moral question: is a human
life more important than that of any nonhuman animal?

The case presents a pointed opportunity for debate between those
who would save a human life at the sacrifice of a baboon and those who
find such salvation morally disgraceful. If it turns out that the use of
baboon livers is scientifically feasible, and setting aside questions of just

distribution, would it be morally conscionable to raise baboons in comfortable surroundings for purposes of human transplant needs?

To answer in the affirmative does not imply that human beings are justified in inflicting pain on sentient animals. It does mean that the painless sacrifice of nonhuman animals for the purpose of saving human lives is acceptable. Arthur L. Caplan challenges those who would place equal moral value on humans and nonhuman animals to consider the neo-Darwinian theorists of the past decade, such as Stephen Jay Gould and Niles Eldredge, who argue that evolution proceeds by leaps and jumps rather than by gradual process and that therefore the gaps between *Homo sapiens* and all other species might be considerable.[33]

Still, I do not defend the use of baboon livers for human patients suffering from irreversible progressive dementia in its more severe stages, for example, advanced Alzheimer's disease. Neither do I defend their use for human beings who lack the potential to develop relational capacities or self-identity. Most people would be disturbed at the idea of sacrificing a baboon to save a human being in the persistent vegetative state. Yet most human beings, on the bases of potential or realized capacities, are fit beneficiaries of baboon livers if in fact benefits can be clearly established. As of yet, benefits remain ambiguous.

When details are available, some may question the particular choice of patient or other clinical-ethical aspects of Starzl's liver transplant. But Starzl has successfully reminded us that the human good remains appropriately the highest good, despite the cultural inroads of anthropomorphism.

Karl Barth understood the gravity of human beings' killing nonhuman animals. He argued convincingly that such killing ought not to be ventured without careful thought about its necessity: "He [man] obviously cannot do this except under the pressure of necessity."[34] We must not exaggerate necessity, or assert it without adequate evidence. Arguably, cruelty or misuse of nonhuman animals fosters a habit of mind that leads to cruelty to fellow human beings.

NOTES

1. National Institutes of Health, *Institutional Administrator's Manual for Laboratory Animal Care and Use*, NIH publication 88-2959 (Bethesda, Md., 1988).

2. Paul Taylor, *Respect for Nature: A Theory of Environmental Ethics* (Princeton, N.J.: Princeton University Press, 1986).

3. Alan Wolfe, "Up from Humanism," *American Prospect* 4 (1991): 112.

4. Willard Gaylin, *Adam and Eve and Pinocchio: On Being and Becoming Human* (New York: Viking, 1990), p. 11.

5. Herbert Pardes, Anne West, and Harold A. Pincus, "Physicians and the Animal Rights Movement," *New England Journal of Medicine* 324 (1991): 1640.

6. *Washingtonian Magazine,* August 1986, p. 115.

7. Peter Singer, *The Expanding Circle: Ethics and Sociobiology* (New York: New American Library, 1981), p. 120.

8. See William Devall and George Sessions, *Deep Ecology: Living as if Nature Mattered* (Los Angeles: Peregrine Smith Books, 1984); Carolyn Merchant, *The Death of Nature: Women, Ecology, and the Scientific Revolution* (San Francisco: Harper and Row, 1983).

9. Padmanabh S. Jaini, *The Jaina Path of Purification,* (Berkeley: University of California Press, 1979).

10. Arne Naess, "The Shallow and the Deep, Long-range Ecology Movement," *Inquiry* 16 (1973): 96; J. Baird Callicott, "Intrinsic Value, Quantum Theory, and Environmental Ethics," *Environmental Ethics* 7 (1985): 257–75.

11. Donald VanDeVeer, "Of Beasts, Persons, and the Original Position," *Monist* 62 (1979): 368–77.

12. Michael Fox, *Returning to Eden: Animal Rights and Human Responsibility* (New York: Viking, 1980).

13. Roger Caras, "We Must Find Alternatives to Animals in Research," *Newsweek,* December 16, 1988.

14. Arne Naess, *Ecology, Community and Lifestyle,* (Cambridge: Cambridge University Press, 1989).

15. James Lovelock, *Gaia: A New Look at Life on Earth,* (London: Oxford University Press, 1974).

16. John Kleinig, *Valuing Life* (Princeton, N.J.: Princeton University Press, 1991), pp. 99, 101.

17. Ibid., p. 101.

18. Michael P. T. Leahy, *Against Liberation: Putting Animals in Perspective* (New York: Routledge, 1992), pp. 219, 226.

19. Michel de Montaigne, "Apology for Raimond Sebond (Man's Presumption and Littleness)," in *The Norton Anthology of World Masterpieces* (New York: W. W. Norton, 1985), pp. 1162–1674.

20. David H. Smith, "Seeing and Knowing Dementia," in Robert H. Binstock, Stephen G. Post, and Peter J. Whitehouse, eds., *Dementia and Aging: Ethics, Values, and Policy Choices* (Baltimore: Johns Hopkins University Press, 1992), chap. 4.

21. Christina Hoff Sommers, "Filial Morality," *Journal of Philosophy* 83, no. 8 (1983): 442.

22. Michael Walzer, *Spheres of Justice: A Defense of Pluralism and Equality* (New York: Basic Books, 1983), pp. 230–231.

23. Edward O. Wilson, *On Human Nature* (Cambridge: Harvard University Press, 1978), p. 158.

24. Stephen J. Pope, "The Order of Love and Recent Catholic Ethics: A Constructive Proposal," *Theological Studies* 52 (1991): 255–288. See J. M. Gustafson, *Ethics and Theology*, vol. 2 of *Ethics from a Theocentric Perspective* (Chicago: University of Chicago Press, 1984), p. 160.

25. Bernard Williams, "A Critique of Utilitarianism," in J. J. C. Smart and Bernard Williams, eds., *Utilitarianism: Pro and Con* (Cambridge: Cambridge University Press, 1973).

26. Carl Cohen, "The Case for the Use of Animals in Biomedical Research," *New England Journal of Medicine* 315 (1986): 867.

27. Peter Singer, *Animal Liberation*, rev. ed. (New York: Avon Books, 1990), p. 6.

28. Nel Noddings, *Caring: A Feminist Approach to Ethics and Moral Education* (Berkeley: University of California Press, 1984), p. 152.

29. Adam Smith, *The Theory of Moral Sentiments*, ed. D. D. Raphael and A. L. Macfie (New York: Oxford University Press, 1976 [original 1759]), p. 216.

30. John Benson, "Duty and the Beast," *Philosophy* 53, no. 206 (1978): 536.

31. R. G. Frey, "Moral Standing, the Value of Lives, and Speciesism," *Between the Species* 8 (1989): 199.

32. L. K. Altman, "2d Transplant Planned Using Liver of Baboon," *New York Times*, September 9, 1992, p. A9.

33. Arthur L. Caplan, "Taking Darwin Seriously," *Medical Humanities Review* 6, no. 2 (1992).

34. Karl Barth, *The Doctrine of Creation*, vol. 3, part 4 of *Church Dogmatics* (Edinburgh: T. & T. Clark, 1961), p. 354.

Index